THE DIGITAL HEALTH SELF

Wellness, Tracking and Social Media

Rachael Kent

BRISTOL
UNIVERSITY
PRESS

First published in Great Britain in 2023 by

Bristol University Press
University of Bristol
1-9 Old Park Hill
Bristol
BS2 8BB
UK
t: +44 (0)117 374 6645
e: bup-info@bristol.ac.uk

Details of international sales and distribution partners are available at bristoluniversitypress.co.uk

British Library Cataloguing in Publication Data
A catalogue record for this book is available from the British Library

ISBN 978-1-5292-1015-6 hardcover
ISBN 978-1-5292-1017-0 ePub
ISBN 978-1-5292-1016-3 ePdf

Cover design: Nicky Borowiec
Front cover image: Composite adapted from (c) phone: pickup/AdobeStock and hand and medical graphics: Tex Vector/AdobeStock with additional icons from Font Awesome
Bristol University Press use environmentally responsible print partners.
Printed and bound in Great Britain by CPI Group (UK) Ltd, Croydon, CR0 4YY

FSC
www.fsc.org
MIX
Paper | Supporting responsible forestry
FSC® C013604

This book is dedicated to the memory of my incredible mother Helen Kent. Your love and wisdom still guides me every day.

– This is for you –

Contents

List of Figures

Note on the figures: We wish to acknowledge that though the figures included in this book are of a low resolution they are integral to the author's content and are the best versions available.

About the Author

Rachael Kent is a world-leading researcher, author and digital health consultant. She is Lecturer in Digital Economy and Society in the Department of Digital Humanities at King's College London, where her research examines the impact of digital technology on mental and physical health.

Dr. Kent is the founder of tech-wellbeing consultancy Dr. Digital Health, providing evidence-based research and strategy for businesses and employees on managing tech saturation, and how tech 'addiction' impacts mental and physical health in everyday professional and personal life. Some of Dr. Kent's clients include the NHS, UK Government, Vivo Barefoot, Paramount and CBS.

Dr. Kent's research regularly appears in press and podcasts including BBC News, *Forbes Magazine*, *Runners World*, *BrainCare*, *Metro UK*, *Heat Magazine*, *Woman and Home Magazine*, *The Daily Mail*, *The Independent*, *MixMag*, *Health and Wellbeing Magazine* and *Glamour Magazine*.

Acknowledgements

The time has come to give thanks to all the many incredible people who have helped and supported me through this challenging but amazing journey of writing my first book. This work is the culmination of 17 years of ideas, research and exploration into how our bodies interact with technology, with its seeds first developing during my undergraduate degree, through my master's, to my PhD and beyond.

There is a huge amount of people to thank for helping this book come into being. If it were not for their guidance and continued support, this book would not exist. In fact, listing everyone would amount to a chapter of this book in and of itself, so I shall make just a few key mentions.

Firstly, I would like to extend a sincere thank you to the whole team at Bristol University Press for their support and guidance with every stage of the writing and editing process – you have been an absolute joy to work with. I would also like to give a special mention to Phoebe Moore for her support during the initial stages of this book proposal. Additionally, I would like to thank the anonymous reviewers for their invaluable feedback that truly shaped the book into a stronger contribution to this field.

I would like to extend a particular mention to a much-valued and trusted colleague and friend, Btihaj Ajana, for her endless support and mentorship. I met Btihaj when she became my PhD supervisor back in 2015, and ever since she has been my absolute advocate! Thank you so much for always being there for me, both as a friend and professionally, providing such sound advice and wisdom. Thank you for all you have enabled for me.

A core part of the research in this book comes from my doctoral research project, for which I would like to thank the European Research Council for funding this work. As a part of the ERC-funded Ego-Media Research Group, I was very fortunate to be surrounded by the incredible expertise of the whole team to guide this doctoral research. To my brilliant Ego-Media colleagues, Max, Clare, Alex, Rob, Becky, Alisa, Charlotte, Stijn, Mikka and my supervisor Leone Ridsdale, I am so grateful to have had all your wisdom to guide me. Thank you for your insights and the opportunities you have all enabled me to be involved in – they have truly enriched this research.

Thank you to my King's College London family, who have been incredible sounding boards and sanity providers! A particular mention goes to the wonderful Photini Vrikki, Simon Tanner, Zeena Feldman and Ashwin Matthew.

There are so many incredible people in my world that I have met and been fortunate enough to work with during this time. My dear friends have shaped my thinking, challenged my ideas, sparked insights and generally been absolute heroes in providing unconditional support, generous advice and at times much-needed comic relief: Kate Longden, Sophie Medlin, Rebecca Saunders, Isla Haslam, Anna Stellardi, Chris Till, Julie Doyle and Rebecca Hiscock.

To my family, James, Megan, Justin, Imogen, Connie, Sara, Ali, Charlotte, Emma, Tim, Anna, Steff, Sri and Peter, thank you for being my forever champions, I appreciate and love you all very much. I would like to give a particular mention to my sister Megan Kent who always provides thought-provoking insights and ideas, is forever an ear or shoulder to cry on when needed, but most importantly is someone I can laugh hysterically with at the nonsense of life – thank you for the respite! To those that are no longer with us – mum, Keith and Chrisi – your love still surrounds us every day.

Lastly, to my Fajri and Monty, the loves of my life, you have kept me going when I thought this day would never come. Thank you for everything.

1

Transformations of Health in the Digital Society

> 'It's hard to quantify what healthy means because there's so many contexts it can apply to.'
>
> (Sophie, final interview, 31, F)

Digital health is both a concept of health management and a daily practice for citizens of the digital society. It is a tool of self-analysis for consumers, a medical framework for health insights, advocated by governments, and public and private healthcare services, as well as, for technology, health, and wellness industries to be capitalised upon. Digital health is now a way of life under the economics of surveillance and platform capitalism, as we all increasingly become autonomous managers of our healthcare via technology, which has only been exacerbated by the COVID-19 pandemic. Digital health is also all the intricate, blurred and hybrid spheres it both silently and overtly occupies within these revolutionary, ethically challenging and problematic intersections. The digital health self, I argue, is the embodiment of evolving with and navigating our everyday lives, traversing between personal lifestyle choice, shifting neoliberal international healthcare and governmental policies, technological advancements and digital capitalism.

The interdisciplinary theoretical framework of this book draws from a wealth of disciplines. The book's analysis of digital health sits at the intersection of several fields: communication studies, media studies, science and technology studies, internet studies, behavioural economics, psychology, sociology and cultural studies, as well as areas of the medical humanities. It provides insights for scholars and students of these fields, and beyond. Its relevance to and application in our current everyday lives also illustrate its significance to those outside of academe – those working in the technology industry, healthcare, both public and private sectors, and the general public for whom managing digital health practices, social media and wellness warrants an increasingly serious consideration in daily life.

This book draws on extensive empirical interview data from two research projects (A: LRS-15/16–2156 and B: MRA-19/20–18193) undertaken before and during the COVID-19 pandemic, which explored individuals' health management via social media and self-tracking apps through a historical analysis of healthcare transformations. It draws upon users' experiences of using digital health technologies and self-tracking tools along with social media to manage their health and wellness in everyday life. Project A undertook empirical ethnographic research over a nine-month period with 14 participants (7 men and 7 women, aged 26–49) who self-selected through a call for participants on Facebook and Instagram, with the selection criteria that they regularly (daily/weekly) share content related to their health and fitness on Facebook and/or Instagram. These participants ranged from the everyday layperson, those who were dieting or training for marathons, to those dealing with illness or disease. The content shared came in the form of self-tracking data from applications (for example, Nike+ or Strava) and devices (for example, Fitbit or Garmin Watch), gym or fitness selfies or more general 'healthy' self-representations such as food photography. The anonymised data collected came from the following sources:

1. two semi-structured interviews (30–45 minutes each), one before and one after the reflexive diary period;
2. bi-monthly guided reflexive diary entries on different days of the week, over a period of three months;
3. screenshots from content shared on Facebook and/or Instagram on the day the reflexive diary was completed (supplied by the participant in the diary and included throughout this book); and
4. textual and thematic analysis of the language used in verbal (interviews) and written (online data and reflexive diaries) formats and screenshots of visual content shared (images and photographs).

Project B undertook one-off interviews with 14 participants (9 men and 5 women, aged 21–50), who self-selected through a call for participants on Facebook and Instagram. No specification of selection criteria was given to enable a wide spectrum of respondents, as interview questions were broadly focused on how any digital technology influenced their mental and physical health in everyday life and how their digital habits had changed since COVID-19. All data presented in this book is anonymised.

Findings from Projects A and B provided insights into the often-neglected perspective of users' direct experience of how technology influences health and wellness. An analysis of these findings identifies how over time these practices shape everyday individual health and wellness behaviours, as well as social media communities' perception of these accounts and experiences, which in turn influence broader socio-cultural conceptualisations, understandings and practices of health (self-) care whilst attending to the evolving technological, political and economic landscape of our everyday life within the digital society. This introductory chapter presents a proposition of what health and digital health have transformed into today. It then provides a brief analytical overview of historical shifts that have impacted and led us to the saturation of digital health and social media for health management. It then moves on to discuss some key concepts, theoretical frameworks and themes that run throughout the book, in particular self-tracking, the role of data and the techno-commercial affordances of social media. Lastly, the chapter provides an overview of the structure of this book and its teachings and findings from the empirical research presented in each of its chapters, from datafication to surveillance to moralism, technology 'addiction', sharing 'healthiness' online and future directions for digital health.

What is digital health?

Health is used in this book as a term to convey, understand and represent human physical and mental wellness, capabilities and capacities. As is illustrative of the neoliberal societies in which we live, I offer a variety of multifaceted conceptualisations of health. The intangible definition of good 'health' can be ascribed to different states of being, which means that health today is regularly maintained by what I term non-traditional healthcare pathways, individual education, self-regulation, self-surveillance and self-tracking. Therefore, 'health' is not used interchangeably in opposition to poor physical or mental health. Rather, 'health' is theoretically framed and interpreted in this book to demonstrate and encompass many aspects of personal lifestyles and wellness: diet, fitness routines, behaviours, the broad relationship we have with our and others' bodies and an overarching sense of personal health identity. Let us now come back to the concept of digital health today. Currently, the World Health Organization (2021: np) understands digital health as

> a broad umbrella term encompassing e-health, as well as developing areas such as the use of advanced computer sciences (for example, in the fields of "big data", genomics and artificial intelligence) – plays an important role in strengthening health systems and public health, increasing equity in access to health services, and in working towards universal health coverage.

I argue that we need to expand our definitions of digital health. Not only can it also be referring to the use of consumer digital technologies, both wearables (for example, Fitbit and Garmin/Strava watch) and apps to track and monitor health (for example, Map My Run or My Fitness Pal), I argue that digital health must also include other digital platforms used in our everyday lives to manage health – most prominently, social media such as Instagram and TikTok – and influencers who provide (sometimes unqualified) mental and physical health, fitness and nutritional guidance and advice. We also need to include and consider the influence of our digital habits, which also impact our mental and physical health in daily life, especially since the COVID-19 pandemic has situated our lives as being increasingly mediated from behind a screen. This has meant, personally, socially and professionally, that there has been a global stagnation of our physicality, being unable to cross borders and making future goals and events challenging to plan and look forward to. This physical stagnation arguably also stagnates the mind, having to deal with the global trauma of living through a pandemic and the residual anxiety, depression and many other mental and physical health impacts. My concern is that globally we will be shaped by these experiences and their impacts; there will be increasing ripple effects upon our mental and physical health for many years to come. Thus, this makes case for further analysis of our digital habits and how they affect daily life, for managing tech saturation, compulsion and even 'addiction' is a contentious daily negotiation for many of us. This book begins this conversation but certainly does not conclude it; more research is needed in this area in coming years. We cannot remove these tools, especially while the global population is living through and beyond COVID-19's impact; thus, effectively managing our digital behaviours in a healthy way becomes an ever present and ever important component of our digital health today.

A review of the existing literature shows that the detrimental effects of health apps has been highlighted by a variety of fields including medicine, psychology, science and technology studies, internet studies and communication studies. Some key findings have demonstrated that weight loss and calorie counting applications (such as MyFitnessPal) have a limited impact on behavioural change, like improving motivation, for example (Lesser et al, 2013) or that their effect is only impactful when used in conjunction with exercise (Spring et al, 2012). The limitations of sleep apps in improving our sleep cycles have been explored (Fage-Butler, 2018; Lupton, 2019), as well as consistent inaccuracies in detecting melanoma across a variety of consumer apps (Wolf et al, 2013). Using health apps and the internet to manage health and self-diagnose may exacerbate the condition of individuals who suffer from anxiety, leading to 'cyberchondria' (Mathes et al, 2018). Broadly, digital technology, smartphones, apps and particularly social media engagement have been consistently linked with negative impacts on mental and physical health (Ajana, 2017, 2021; Kent, 2018, 2020, 2021; Lupton, 2019; Feldman and Goodman, 2021), and where this book contributes to this developing field is in exploring these claims from the everyday perspective of the individual. The research presented in this book uniquely contributes to this field by examining how self-tracking and social media apps impact both mental and physical health from an empirical perspective of the individual and how this influences health management and behavioural change from a long-term perspective.

What this book calls for and presents through this empirical data is a reconceptualisation of what digital health practically means in individuals' everyday lives. In this vein, I consider how following an influencer's lifestyle guidance can also be considered a component of one's digital health practices today, as much as their daily Fitbit tracking. In addition, how these self-monitoring and scrolling practices might become a part of an individual's daily tech habits, and in turn their 'addictive' or compulsive nature, must also be included as part of one's 'digital health'. From adjusting your physical movements, to capture more step counts on your Fitbit, to being unable to stop scrolling social media accounts can all now be considered as part of the arsenal of digital economy practices that impact one's health, mentally or physically – and in many instances both! Therefore, I propose a more inclusive and expansive definition of digital health in the digital society of 2023, comprising five different elements:

(1) wearable and self-tracking health apps (Fitbit, Strava, or MapMyRun),
(2) telehealth and telemedicine
(3) digital platforms for health information (WebMD, AI Chatbots, Babylon Health),
(4) social media (such as Instagram) and influencer culture for following 'health guidance' (Kent, 2018, 2020, 2021), and
(5) digital habits, our daily relationship with digital devices and how we manage everyday technological saturation.

Digital health today refers to both traditional and non-traditional healthcare pathways and management mediated by technology, which include personal health tracking and monitoring via consumer or medical devices, technological tools for clinical intervention from our medical providers, digital platforms (including social media and influencers) for accessing and navigating health (mis)information and guidance, the inferences and profiling generated from the data mining of our digital behaviours and interactions across the internet, and our daily habits with our digital devices.

Digital health is never neutral, as these platforms, practices, tools and interventions are regularly capitalised upon by digital capitalists, particularly from the technology, health and wellness industries. This is why this book's title 'the digital health self' is proposed as a new concept and terminology to encapsulate and attend to these influences and navigations; therefore, as mentioned at the very beginning of this chapter, my definition of the digital health self is as follows:

> The digital health self is the embodiment of evolving with and navigating our everyday lives, traversing between personal lifestyle choice and wellness goals, shifting neoliberal international healthcare and governmental policies, technological advancements, under digital capitalism.

Digital health and its history

The welfare state

This section provides a historical contextualisation of health tracking and public health communication from the post-World War Two development of the British National Health Service (NHS) in 1948, through the birth of neoliberalism, until today's individualising practices of digital health tracking and quantification of bodies. As a result of these three phases of public health quantification of bodies, encompassing the socio-economic, cultural and political shifts since 1948, combined with the development and wide adoption of digital health and self-quantifying technologies, the changing landscape has had dramatic implications for shifting who is responsible for maintaining 'good' health. After the quantification strategies of the food and consumer goods rationing of World War Two, the United Kingdom presented the state as being responsible for the health and wellbeing of its population by developing the NHS in 1948. In turn, the UK welfare state was born. With the birth of the NHS, doctors and medical staff were seen as purveyors of health expertise, seen as 'medical prestige' in the eyes of the public (Seale, 2003). Social determinants of health were identified as influencers in the causation and containment of disease. This shifted citizens from consumers to patients: part of a healthcare system that invoked feelings of inclusion, unity and support, with the NHS's clinical expertise as the safeguarder of UK public health.

The birth of neoliberalism and healthism

The second phase of the transformation describes the dramatic public health promotion and policy shifts from the 1960s onwards until the global recession of 2008. These shifts included a move away from the inclusive welfare state ideologies towards promoting individualised health management under neoliberal governments around the world. The dominance of neoliberal rationalities over public health was further cemented during the economic and unemployment crises of the 1970s and 1980s (Harvey, 2005), putting the economy before the needs of the people (Brown, 2005) and prioritising open, competitive and unregulated markets. This process created a shift from the classic liberal values of the welfare state as a supporter and facilitator of public health towards neoliberal practices, which included the privatisation of public institutions and the self. Neoliberalism, in response to the global financial crisis of 2008, has resulted in the resolution of many countries to 'cut back (…) the welfare state and public spending (…) The issue today is not limited to a single country, as neoliberalism is an international, even global, phenomenon' (Crouch, 2011: viii). This global neoliberal rationality positions the citizen as a consumer self-regulating to make the 'right' ethical decisions for the management of individual self-care. Within neoliberalism we also see shifts towards 'responsibilisation', which is a term from the literature of governmentality referring to 'the process whereby subjects are rendered individually responsible for a task which previously would have been the duty of another – usually a state agency – or would not have been recognized as a responsibility at all' (Wakefield and Fleming, 2009: 277). The cultural and political shifts towards neoliberalism led to a form of health promotion on the part of both the state and commercial business, which was characterised by practices of 'healthism' (Crawford, 1980) and responsibilisation.

> Healthism is defined here as the preoccupation with personal health as a primary (…) focus for the definition and achievement of well-being; a goal which is to be attained primarily through the modification of life styles, with or without therapeutic help (…) For the healthiest, solution rests within the individual's determination to resist culture, advertising, institutional and environmental constraints, disease agents, or, simply, lazy or poor personal habits. (Crawford, 1980: 386)

Healthism presented lifestyle correction that is achievable only via practices of individual responsibility (Leichter, 1997). Good living, in 'healthism', is dependent upon individuals making healthy choices (Crawford, 1980: 378) and becoming entrepreneurial subjects seeking out the best self-care for health. I see here how such a restructuring and dismantling of social and economic spheres 'figures and produces citizens as individual entrepreneurs and consumers whose moral autonomy is measured by their capacity for "self-care"' (Brown, 2005; 694). Through the concept of neoliberal 'governmentality' (Foucault, 1979a) the regulatory activity both of the self and of the external influences was advocated by healthcare policy and the media, shaping public beliefs and behaviours towards individual regulation and self-maintenance. One of these strategies of self-responsibilisation was the 'privileging' of 'good' health and lifestyle choice with inherent victim-blaming inclinations despite socio-economic determinations of disease in medicine (Lupton, 2013a). The development of disease and ill health has long been viewed as a consequence of an individual lack of self-discipline and intrinsic moral failing (Mennel et al, 1992; Brandt and Rozin, 1997). Sufferers and 'victims' of ill health and disease would therefore be positioned by healthcare promotion and policy as being irresponsible and would subsequently be blamed for poor health management. This discourse argued that irrespective of whether you are dealing with chronic disease or minor ailment you are responsible for managing that on a day-to-day basis (Lorig and Holman, 2003). A refusal to engage in healthy behaviours or to actively manage ill health, according to Lorig and Holman (2003: 1), reflects a poor 'management style':

> Unless one is totally ignorant of healthful behaviors it is impossible not to manage one's health. The only question is how one manages. The issue of self-management is especially important for those with chronic disease, where only the patient can be responsible for his or her day-to-day care over the length of the illness. For most of these people, self-management is a lifetime task.

'Good' health and a healthy body are no longer simply considered in opposition to ill health but have become demonstrative of economic and social factors and self-discipline, thus further cementing ill health within a moral sphere. To further extend Lorig and Holman's (2003) argument, it is not just sufferers of chronic conditions but the everyday layperson who now embodies this dominant discourse. Health self-management, when not enacted effectively, becomes tied to personal blame (and shame) over lack of personal responsibility and poor health management.

Digital self-care and COVID-19 pandemic

The third and most recent phase of health transformations has evolved since the global recession and financial crash of 2008, with its accompanying global austerity, increasing privatisation of public health services and the pervasive promotion and adoption of digital health technologies, as a direct impact of our current digital society. This has reached its culmination to date with COVID-19 contact tracing apps. The novel coronavirus now globally known as COVID-19 was first identified in December 2019 and quickly grew into a global pandemic affecting at least 223 countries, with 439 million confirmed cases and sadly 5.9 million confirmed deaths worldwide (World Health Organization, 2021). Governments around the world have attempted to manage the spread through a variety of digital health and surveillance tools (for example, China's 'Health Code'). In the United Kingdom, the government attempted to manage the spread of COVID-19 through NHS public health initiatives such as 'Test and Trace' (testing for COVID-19 through home testing or walk-in sites) and the NHS COVID-19 app (UK Government, 2021), which provides users with contact tracing services, local area alerts and geo-tagging venue check-ins. Similar technological initiatives have been developed internationally in an attempt to reduce the spread of COVID-19, further expanding the bounds of what digital health means to citizens and state and how the tracking and quantification of bodies are increasingly normalised in a digital society responding to a global pandemic. To give an indication of how pervasive the digital health market has become, the commercial market alone was valued at $106 billion in 2019 and is projected to grow to a global market value of $605 billion by 2025 (Statistica, 2021), which will have dramatic implications for health management globally, especially given these statistics were projected prior to COVID-19.

The COVID-19 pandemic has placed pressures on the general public not only to gain a level of expertise of medical health management knowledge but also to responsibilise their citizenship in ways we have never yet seen in global public health. Through the underpinning of the current pervasive digital society, we see a multitude of ways citizens have become lay experts of viral illness, navigating tsunamis of information and misinformation online to equip themselves in attempts to keep themselves, their family, friends and colleagues safe (Kent, 2020, 2021). To ensure avoidance of doubt, I would like to clarify that 'lay experts/expertise' is used throughout this book not as a labelling of inferior intellectual insight to qualified experts or influencers, professional athletes for example, but to refer to those users and general public who draw upon 'experiential knowledge':

> [This] refers to the ultimate source of patient-specific knowledge—the often implicit, lived experiences of individual patients with their bodies and their illnesses as well as with care and cure. Experiential knowledge arises when these experiences are converted, consciously or unconsciously, into a personal insight that enables a patient to cope with individual illness and disability. (Caron-Flinterman et al, 2005: 2575)

This book broadens this definition and refers to lay experts as not limited to the patient or healthcare context but also to the general population who, in response to COVID-19, have armed themselves with related healthcare guidance to educate themselves, as well as to users who turn to digital platforms and social media for health guidance. 'Lay expertise' identification, then, in this research is illustrated by any practices related to those individuals gaining experiential knowledge, which refers to how these users turn their experiences into understanding, as well as patients or those suffering with illness, to explain the motivation to gain health and virus-related information for self-care and wellbeing. When the accumulation of knowledge or the 'communal body of knowledge exceeds the boundaries of individual experiences' (Caron-Flinterman et al, 2005: 2577), this has been referred to as 'experiential expertise' (Meijer et al, 1993; Van der Schaaf and Oderwald, 1999); however, for coherence this book considers this stage as a part of the process of gaining 'lay expertise' for personal safeguarding and wellness.

Citizens increasingly shared these journeys on social media, a performance of visible optimal health practices in pandemic life, including invisible illnesses like COVID-19 (Kent, 2021). This became a widely adopted practice on Instagram, Facebook, TikTok, Twitter and WeChat during COVID-19 lockdowns and ongoing restrictions (Kent, 2021). Through exhibiting aesthetically 'Insta-worthy' lockdowns and lifestyle restrictions under COVID-19 we move from 'FOMO' (fear of missing out) to 'toxic productivity' (the fear of not being perceived as productive), not only inside the home with the increasing digital mediatisation and blurring of labour and leisure in the pandemic but also with respect to productive health management and risk reduction individually as well as collectively for public health safety. Showcasing to your social media community you were conforming to restrictions and keeping healthy and safe became a signifier of a productive, happy and successful lockdown and citizenship practice (Kent, 2020). So much so, the stigmatisation of contracting COVID-19 in the early days of the pandemic (Kent, 2020) became ascribed to once archaic discourses of irresponsibility and immoral behaviour being linked with ill health that are still prevalent today (Kent, 2021).

A long-term implication of the increasing adoption of consumer health apps since 2010, now exacerbated by surveillance cultures of contact tracing during COVID-19, is that the quantification and health tracking of bodies have become a normalised discourse in international public health promotion as well as individual citizenship and patient practices. Free market principles have reigned over international public health discourse for many decades, seeing health as no longer binary to illness but as a practice of individual self-quantification and self-care, which has only been further intensified by the COVID-19 pandemic. International public health strategies promote the use of digital health and contact tracing technologies, thus positioning citizens as entrepreneurial subjects, adopting extensive technological measures in an attempt to measure, monitor and 'optimise' health, which increasingly normalises the everyday quantification and digital monitoring of health and bodies.

Self-tracking and social media as digital health tools

Self-tracking technologies and social media platforms enable a variety of ways to represent 'health'. What makes self-tracking new in the context of this book is its digitisation and subsequent engagement with performativity on social media and how this influences everyday health behaviours. Through the sharing of self-tracking data on social media, self-monitoring of the body is extended into the communities' gaze. This book is concerned with the practice of knowing one's body and 'health' through using these apps and devices to self-regulate the fit and idealised 'healthy' subject, as well as the promotion of such lifestyles through the comparative and competitive practices embedded within social media (Facebook and Instagram). The emerging body of research around mobile devices, in particular 'wearables', has addressed the significance of geo-locative devices and apps and healthcare data repositories (Oudshoorn, 2011; Mort et al, 2013). These practices are, however, no longer confined to volunteering individuals (with all the subjectifying self-regulatory responsibilisation this entails) but also includes employers and insurance companies, who advocate and even incentivise their use within corporate wellness schemes and healthcare package deals they offer to employees and customers (Olson and Tilley, 2014; Moore et al, 2018; Till, 2018). There has been extensive research exploring the use of self-tracking technologies in multiple settings, such as work and insurance schemes, schools, self-quantification/tracking communities and leisure pursuits (Lupton, 2014, 2016a; Rettberg, 2014, 2018; Fotopoulou and O'Riordan, 2016; Ajana, 2017, 2018b; Goodyear et al, 2017; Moore, 2017; Kristensen and Prigge, 2018; Moore et al, 2018; Ruffino, 2018; Spiller et al, 2018; Till, 2018). However, there is a paucity of research on the use of these technologies in representations of 'health' on social media in relation to how these curated health identities affect users' health behaviours in their daily lives.

Neoliberalism and new materialism

Neoliberalism, as explored in this chapter so far, has been understood as a rationality advocated by state institutions, prioritising free market principles and 'the dominance of public life by the giant corporation' (Crouch, 2011: viii) over the body, which advocates that individual responsibility for health management is enacted through the adoption of consumer heath technologies. As Moore and Robinson (2016: 2776) observe, neoliberalism can be understood 'as an affective regime exposing a risk of assumed subordination of bodies to technologies'. As a mode of governance then, neoliberalism is a political rationality that has become a pervasive tool to dictate and promote self-transformation of health (through the use of technology) as the continual lifestyle goal for individuals, citizens and patients. The tensions and dualisms between the body and mind in being 'productive' to obtain an optimising state of health can be understood through the lens of 'new materialism', which 'sets out to approach studies of life and knowledge in new ways that better reflect contemporary circumstances where survival is biological, and production is often virtual' (Moore, 2017: np).

This conceives of the mind as having control over matter, or indeed culture can be considered as dominant over nature (Van der Tuin and Dolphijn, 2010: 156), and the mind having control over the body. Therefore, new materialism offers ways of understanding how the assemblage of humans and technology has a liveliness, whereby all types of matter are an organising and agential experience (Moore and Robinson, 2016). As Moore and Robinson (2016: 2780) astutely identify, in a neoliberal society self-tracking and social media sharing of the body and digital health self

> transgresses the mind–body split; however, it also places the mind firmly in control. In this binary, the mind determines rational knowledge and quantification. The body (and 'spirit') is a passive object of this process, subject to being improved, whether they like it or not. The body has no agency of its own accord. It also creates contradictions because the Cartesian split is maintained even while recognising the inseparability of body and mind.

Using this perspective and recognition of how individuals attempt to manage their body and perceive it as malleable through the productive mind via digital technology, this book explores and identifies how human subjectivity is structurally embodied (Braidotti, 2005: 158; Moore and Robinson, 2016). The self becomes 'managed', in 'both her subjectivity and the outer world, (…) [reproducing] the Cartesian trope of the subordination of (risky) body to (rational) mind' (Moore, 2017: np). In this book then, I examine the dominant role neoliberal ideology plays in the mind of individuals, advocating governance and control over the body through technological intervention – the true embodiment of the digital health self. The capacity to transform is advocated through these political rationalities contending that better health is achievable only through optimising and moulding the matter of the body via the dominant, powerful and assertive mind of the individual. The increase in the number of neoliberal governments has involved 'a reorganisation of the powers of the state, with the devolution of many responsibilities for the management of human health and reproduction that, across the twentieth century had been responsibility of the formal apparatus of government: devolving these to quasi-autonomous regulatory bodies' (Rose, 2007: 3). Consumer self-tracking devices can then be considered techno-deterministic and techno-utopian in their promotion of the idea that data capture is the best method to improve health and their tools are the best available, whereby technology is seen as having the ability to transform individual health and mould bodily matter into optimal performance. In addition, these perspectives provide certain ways of knowing what data is, why it is important, who gets to interpret it and to what ends. I shall continue this conversation in the following section.

The role of data

The role of data in digital health practices is often the key motivator for engagement in consumer self-tracking devices. Neff and Nafus (2016: 189) argue that the 'line between data and ourselves is where we choose to draw it'. This book, however, argues that users do not always have this choice, nor are these distinctions clear, especially with regard to data surveillance and privacy. As we have seen with the increasing adoption of both self-tracking and social media platforms, users voluntarily engage with these platforms and devices and willingly give up personal data; as soon as the data enters the human and non-human assemblage, whether this be online or offline, the proprietor is no longer solely the user who generated it. To unpack this in comparative medical terms, our personal data held by doctors and clinicians in traditional healthcare settings such as a GP surgery or hospital is afforded protection (Data Protection Act, 1998). Personal data uploaded onto digital health devices, applications and social media (Nike +, My Fitness Pal, Google, Facebook and so on) is collected and sold on to advertisers and marketers (Shahini, 2012). Moore (2017: np) argues further and conceives that 'capitalism, as the current global political economic model within which we live, is becoming a system of increasingly empty selves, subject to unending capitalist social reproduction, where data simply confirms the order it has already prefabricated'. Thus, the seductive feature of these devices and technologies for laypeople is the promise of connectivity as well as health optimisation, community support and advice. However, as many of these platforms and applications are free to use, privacy is perceived by users as the ideological and practical 'trade-off' for using 'free' services. The participants in the research projects I refer to throughout this book frequently viewed data mining not as an invasion of their privacy but rather as an acceptable practice that is an intricate part of their use of these technologies, the re-articulation and representation of the body and self through their use and, most interestingly, useful visual tools to share health-related behaviours on social media as a performance for the communities' gaze. Therefore, in accordance with Moore (2017: np), the ideal self-tracker is

> (a) one who cognitively recognises that the mind and the machine must join forces to control physical movement and the affective experience or emotional responses to work [and health management], (b) someone who knows that their non-cognitive self is in constant need of self-improvement, and so, (c) is perpetually imperfect.

Individuals using digital health technologies, sharing data and health-related content on social media, become both subjects and subjected; they are constructed and conceived. These new subjectivities, which emerge through self-tracking technologies and data sharing, have been termed 'datafication'

(Mayer-Schönberger and Cukier, 2013: 30) and 'dataveillance' (van Dijck, 2014: 198). This reflects Hjorth's (2011) and Allen's (2008) observations that the everyday user may not reflect upon the role of such data collection in wider systemic and political terms. Jose van Dijck (2014: 198) defines 'dataism' as the 'widespread belief in the objective quantification and potential tracking of all kinds of human behaviour and sociality through online media technologies'. Immaterial and de-corporealised representations of the body restructure our lived experience (Ajana, 2013; Lupton, 2014; Moore and Robinson, 2016; Sherman, 2016; Moore, 2017), for, as Kristensen and Prigge (2018: 44) highlight, 'the subject doing the measuring, is also "delivering" that material to be measured, interpreting the data and acting on these', thus contributing to a continually evolving, involved and expanding relationship with data and how it is experienced. Therefore, this construction of a digital health self entails a new conception of lived experience, where the self is known through data and the data simultaneously informs the self, both in online sharing and in offline behaviours. This book, however, is concerned not only with the quantified representations of the body and health but also with other health-related, at times qualitative, forms of representations, which I have previously referred to as the 'health self' (Kent, 2018: 62). Therefore, this book, and my proposition of the 'digital health self', encompasses and refers to many different types of bodily, health and fitness representations enabled through the convergence of self-tracking apps, devices and social media in the digital society.

Making sense of our health through digital technology

Self-tracking and digital health sensors, computers, wearables and other forms of new technology extend human powers into digitally quantifiable (Lupton, 2012b) as well as qualitative formats and dualisms between the mind and the body. At the same time, they demonstrate the shift from a public welfare state responsibility for health towards individualised and self-responsibilising practices of health self-care within neoliberal societies (Harvey, 2005; Hey, 2005; Aguirre et al, 2006; Tritter, 2009; Crouch, 2011; Lupton, 2013; Davies, 2015, 2016). As Cederstrom and Spicer (2015: 5) argue, wellness is now not a choice but a 'moral obligation', and the same can be understood of health management in current neoliberal societies. Many digital health technologies hold within their capacities a 'one size fits all' model of health management and self-care. As Buyx and Prainsack (2012: 82) explain: 'research in epigenetics has shown that some environmental influences, such as the consumption of particular foods, can change the way genes are switched on or off, leading to a situation where the social is effectively folded into the genetic and vice versa.' This means that it is increasingly difficult to differentiate between genetic, non-genetic and lifestyle influences upon individual health, which ensures that 'against this backdrop of lack of knowledge and empirical research, the notion of what we can be held accountable for is clearly a moving target' (Buyx and Prainsack, 2012: 82). This 'moving target' of health improvement raises socio-cultural issues in the context of everyday digital health management and self-care, with increasing pressures for citizens and patients to attempt the arbitrary goal of 'optimal' health, which is often intangible and may be unachievable; hence, the health goals cannot be met. This book, therefore, explores the relationship between power and knowledge and how it is diffused in politicised practices advocated and enforced within self-tracking technologies and self-representation on social media, within the cycle of health optimisation that never ends. How can we be satisfied with working towards a health goal when the goalpost keeps moving, via the sensationalist and ambiguous currencies of 'optimisation' and 'wellness'?

Lupton (2006: 94–95) argues that Foucault and his derivatives often 'neglect examination of the ways that hegemonic medical discourses and practices are variously taken up, negotiated or transformed by members of the lay population in their quest to maximise their health status and avoid physical distress and pain'. Therefore, this book addresses this gap in research through an empirical ethnographic study of users' experiences of self-tracking technologies and their relationship with their health identity, as they strive towards self-betterment and health optimisation. This empirical research is significant, as it renders the arguments of Foucault (and his derivatives) less abstract by providing valuable insights into how laypeople negotiate and navigate dominant neoliberal and medical discourses in their everyday lives through an examination of individual strategies for the management of health. This book, therefore, examines the increasingly neoliberal political, socio-economic and cultural shifts that promote 'a view of people whose ability to prosper is unrelated to traditional features of survival under capitalist conditions, such as an income and the ability to feed bodies' (Moore, 2017: np). Rather, I see a promotion of the move towards individual and self-responsibilising health practices in enabling optimal bodies, afforded and encouraged by self-tracking technologies, the corporations that market their revolutionising potentials and the state. This research conducts a critical analysis of how users mediate relationships between these technologies and their health practices, with self-tracking technologies being considered a lifestyle tool to aid and enable health decisions. Wellness and healthism are key ideologies throughout my analysis, focusing upon the persistent prioritisation of health or certain representations of 'healthy' lifestyles and behaviours for these users. These comparative and competitive practices can be understood as what Strava (2015, cited in Lupton, 2016a: 24) terms 'social fitness'. This book, therefore, explores how these technologies influence and enable certain self-representations of health and health identity and how such practices of self-representation within online communities (Facebook and Instagram) enable ways of experiencing and viewing one's own body and health in relation to others.

Whereas biometrics have become shadowed by a dystopian surveillant discourse (Magnet, 2011; Ajana, 2012, 2013), digital health and self-tracking technologies through health promotion strategies advocated by the neoliberal states and the corporations who market their benefits have until very recently evaded such critique. Indeed, they have primarily been promoted as revolutionary tools for health betterment. Lupton (2013f: 14) articulates this as a 'data utopian discourse on the possibilities and potential of big data, metricisation and algorithmic calculation for healthcare'. Advocacy for the use of digital health technologies is also increasingly evident in international policy (Rich and Miah, 2017), as these technologies are seen to provide 'cost-effective preventative solutions to rising levels of obesity, sedentary behaviour and associated non-communicable diseases' (World Health Organization, 2011; HM Government, 2015; Goodyear et al, 2017: 1–2). The promotion of such digital health technologies through such health promotion campaigns often disregards the social, cultural and political dimensions of their use (Lupton, 2014), in particular, how individual responsibility, management and enactment of 'healthy' lifestyles become entwined with consumer culture and free market neoliberal rationalities. Poor health or a lack of health management is a threat not only to individual health but also to society, 'shifting the focus from an unhealthy activity to an unhealthy individual'; therefore, 'when health becomes an ideology, the failure to conform becomes a stigma' (Cederstrom and Spicer, 2015: 4). Conformity, along with control, therefore, is often presented as self-responsibilising empowerment of wellness. Neff and Nafus (2016) argue that these practices are enabling enhanced knowledge of the self and body. However, this book critically examines, through empirical data of self-tracking users, how these practices can be identified more as an unknown in what they provide for their users (Dyer, 2016). It will critique these promised discourses and will challenge what these 'new intimacies of surveillance' (Berson, 2015: 40) and new technological interrogations of the body actually provide the user with. This reflexive and cyclical process challenges the notion of the self, as 'a bounded entity, with a fixed and stable ontology' (Kristensen and Ruckenstein, 2018: 4). Rather, new forms of visualisation and communication emerge from these identity formations (Ruckenstein, 2017) through the unknown (Dyer, 2016) and 'the interplay between self-tracking practices and wider healthcare discourses and emergent strategies' (Ajana, 2017: 2). Kristensen and Ruckenstein (2018: 3–4) understand these human–technology relationships as forming a '"laboratory of the self" framing self-tracking and associated human–technology interactions as metrics-enhanced self-experimentation and discovery'. Self-tracking was once framed through academic literature and the corporations who promoted them as enabling 'healthier' bodies, with the mind–body relational sphere being frequently omitted in earlier analyses. More recent work has attended to this continuum. For example, Pink and Fors (2017: 2) consider self-tracking technologies to mediate 'people's tacit ways of being in the world', paying attention to the intimate forged relational modalities between technology, the body and the mind. Moore and Robinson (2016) argue how quantified self-practices and self-tracking technologies rely upon the ontological premise of Cartesian dualism with the mind being dominant over the body. Therefore, framing and understanding self-tracking practices as a 'laboratory of the self' provide a holistic examination of these processes of 'objectification and subjectification, framing new possibilities as well as imperatives for self-exploration and self-improvement' (Kristensen and Ruckenstein, 2018: 4). The use of self-tracking technologies, therefore, leads to the metrification of 'health' (Ajana, 2018b), as well as the curation of 'health(y)' identities through the 'share-ability' of these metrics on social media. The role of data and these technologies in shaping our understandings of our bodies and our 'health' highlights the discourses of self-governance and self-discipline that exist within cultures of self-tracking. Additionally, these movements and cultures purvey that the characteristics of agility, continual transformation and change are now a pervasive part of being in neoliberal society of control (Deleuze, 1992; Moore, 2017).

Social media and performing the digital health self

This book examines the use by individuals of self-tracking and social media platforms as ethnographic sites for health management, which enables a critical analysis of the subjects' self-representations. The practice of using social media therefore 'requires a critical approach to context creation; (…) participation in social networking entails both the production of one's own self-representation and the acceptance that one may be represented by others' (Thumin, 2012: 149). This book, therefore, defines and conceptualises social media platforms, in particular Facebook and Instagram, as performative spheres for the construction of identity including the social, cultural and psychological aspects of behaviour through communication and surveillance technologies. These ethnographic sites and the empirical analysis enable interrogation of the online representations, offline realities and lived experiences of these individuals. However, it must be highlighted that the ethnography in this book does not attend to analysis of these platforms (Facebook and Instagram) of self-representation themselves. Rather, the focus centres on the participants' use of and engagement with these platforms for their own representational and surveillant needs. The online data captured (screenshots) was supplied by the participants of their self-tracked or health-related content shared on Facebook and Instagram. This book provides a unique contribution to the expanding field of self-tracking technologies through its analysis of participants' processes and practices related to using these technologies to represent their health identities and how such performances, under the online communities' gaze, affect their health behaviours and practices offline. As Kristensen and Ruckenstein (2018: 2) articulate: 'These collaborations (…) mediate and modify human presence and perception, behaviour and decision making', enabling participants to generate new ways of seeing themselves through such self-representational performances on social media. This further shapes 'self-understanding and self-expression, suggesting a vision of technology that in its concrete materiality influences not only selves, bodies and socialities but also communication and learning' (Kristensen and Ruckenstein, 2018: 2). Therefore, my analysis explores how these technologies mediate users' perceptions of themselves and their personal actions. Once 'health'-related content is shared, this analysis then examines how participants conceptualise 'health'-related experience individually and through the gaze of others watching in their social media communities.

Self-representation, in a neoliberal age, is often achieved through individualising practices and a sharing of statistics or lifestyles. This book defines the self-representation practices enabled through self-tracking and social media platforms through the lens of Goffman's (1959) work, which identifies self-presentation as a performance. When we historicise the internet, we can begin with the argument that it holds within its processes and practices the commercial exploitation of leisure as a means for controlling personal and collective identity (Wallace, 1999; Jakala and Berki, 2004). Whereas before writers published historical narratives and constructed cultural and social histories, with the affordances of web 2.0 and in particular social media, users are now able to individually construct their own. Instagram describes itself as 'a community of more than 800 million who capture and share the world's moments on the service' (Instagram , 2018). Facebook similarly identifies itself as a platform that 'give[s] people the power to build community and bring the world closer together' (Facebook , 2018). Maslow (1987) argues that being part of a group or community fulfils part of a basic human need to belong, identifying why individuals may feel a desire to join and maintain a presence and self-representation within social networks and online communities. We now speak with these platforms through representational mediations of self.

Commodification of sociality and sharing

When unpacking the production of the self, through self-representation online as a conscious process that seeks to legitimise an original or authentic persona, social media users are attempting to construct an idealised self through careful assembling. van Dijck likens the construction of online personas to the construction of personal 'brands': 'Promoting and branding of the self has (…) become a normalised, accepted, phenomena in ordinary people's lives' (van Dijck, 2013a: 3). We can consider interactions online and the types of self-presentations projected as a form of self-branding and in turn a commodification of social ties. In this process, 'strategically appealing to followers becomes a carefully calculated way to market oneself as a commodity in response to employment uncertainty' (Marwick and boyd, 2010: 6; see also Lair et al, 2005; Hearn, 2008). However, this book is not concerned with analysing users of social media who gain commercially from constructing and sharing self-representational health content, known as 'influencers' (Freberg et al, 2010: 1). It deals with the general public who, through sharing content, may without premeditation commodify their self and become a 'micro-celebrity' of their own lives (Marwick and boyd, 2010: 114). This 'micro-celebrity' is a form of personal branding and strategic self-commodification through performance in consideration to the (imagined) audiences online (Marwick and boyd, 2010). Personal branding online becomes synonymous with 'authenticity', often without recognition that 'authenticity' is very much a social construct (Sternberg, 1998). These types of self-presentation are conceived with thought to the expression one 'gives' and the expression one 'gives off' (Goffman, 1959). Therefore, the impression that the user attempts to 'give off' and perform may be related to the considerations of the group requiring certain types of expression (Goffman, 1959). The 'imagined' audience or expected community surveillance mediate this self-presentation: 'Individuals learn how to manage tensions between public and private, insider and outsider, and frontstage and backstage performances' (Marwick and boyd, 2010: 17). However, we cannot always ensure that the presentation we attempt to 'give off' is received as intended:

> Knowing that the individual is likely to present himself in a light that is favourable to him, the others may divide what they witness into two parts: a part that is relatively easy for the individual to manipulate at will, being chiefly his verbal assertions and a part in regard to which he seems to have little concern or control being chiefly derived from the expressions he gives off. (Goffman, 1959: 139)

The splitting of perceptions within social media, the online community, audience or group must be acknowledged. Goffman understands this as something of an information game: 'a potentially infinite cycle of concealment, discovery, false revelation and rediscovery' (1959: 140), as an attempt to manage and maintain the perception the user 'gives off'.

Over extended periods of time and through aging and evolving with these technologies,

> users may release more 'social' and personal data than they would like, but it also gives them an instrument to carefully craft their public profile. The fine line between what has been called 'authentic' and 'idealised' (or inauthentic) self-promotion requires a precarious balancing act (…) which users are not always aware of or are not always good at. (van Dijck, 2013b: 211)

For example, 'reputations on social media are treated as an individual responsibility, while in practice exceeding individual control' (Trottier, 2012: 321) in relation to data mining and invasions of privacy, as well as algorithmic sorting and visibility of content.

Little is often understood by the everyday user of how algorithmic sorting works in each social media platform or self-tracking technology. It is important for users to recognise that visibility is not transparent or impartial. Rather, it is linked to a series of small actions, and the connections between users and their value are attributed to these actions by algorithms and their personalised data economies. Barriers to understanding how content is situated and organised still exist for some users with regard to how news feeds or content streams of Facebook, Instagram and self-tracking technologies are algorithmically fabricated. It can therefore be asked how algorithms create visibility for the networked image, status update or content and why this is important for networked sociality, communication and self-representational practices. We are creating a representation of ourselves on these platforms, which places users as subjects whose visibility is algorithmically informed and curated; arguably, these filters are not an arbiter of truth but a barrier to authenticity. Therefore, these socio-technological affordances and forms of algorithmic sorting can be seen as a form of disciplinary control and an extension of the bio-political: the identification and regulation of life logging and governance of the self. As this is achieved by 'forcing users to encode their information homogenously, it is easier to automatically detect patterns of behaviour and manipulate them' (van Dijck, 2013b: 206). Here we can identify how the technological affordances and functionality of platforms regulate and discipline certain information as well as communication and sociality, which is then commercially mined: 'Platform owners are interested in standardisation as well as customisation; if personal data are inserted and presented uniformly, it is easier for advertisers to mass-customise and personalise their marketing strategies, while real-time statistics help them keep track of their success' (van Dijck, 2013b: 206). These platforms, therefore, blur the lines between sociality and consumerism, whereby algorithms can be identified as coded quantifications of sociality to enable both sincere and capitalist connections (Beer, 2008, 2009; van Dijck, 2013a, 2013b).

Book structure

This introductory chapter discussed the research objectives and findings and provided the empirical foundations for this book as well as the key theoretical, socio-cultural, economic and political transformations in which this research is situated. It then moved on to contextualise the theoretical and thematic frameworks that are used throughout the book to help analyse this phenomenon of self-tracking and social media practices and sharing of individual health and wellness in everyday life. I now provide a brief overview of the structure of this book, as its chapters take a logical analysis using these aforementioned frameworks, highlighting the key practices and cultures of the digital health self in today's digital society.

Chapter 2, 'Understanding Our Bodies through Datafication', analyses the techno-commercial infrastructures of self-tracking and social media as processes of datafication, whereby all data can now be conceived as a form of health data through digital phenotyping. I attend to the behavioural economics and choice architecture of these devices and gamification tactics such as nudging and engagement tools, as well as the coercive elements of using these technologies in everyday life. I conclude the chapter by explaining how acquiring quantifications of health (such as 'likes' on health and social media apps) provides a currency of perceived emotional nourishment and physical motivation for these users.

Chapter 3, 'Surveillance Cultures of the Digital Health Self', explores the many ways in which the body is voluntarily and unknowingly surveilled by self-tracking and social media platforms. I identify the ambiguous goal of health betterment as providing no bounds for users, much like the surveillance from the self, community, tech company and the state knows no visible bounds in these data-sharing and data-mining spheres. I explore the process of identifying unexpected surveillance from unseen others and its impact upon what users share or conceal over time on social media. I conclude this chapter by identifying the mechanised patterns of controlling and managing the body through inputs (consumption) and outputs (exercise/energy expenditure) as a surveillance-focused health management tool for users when using self-tracking and social media platforms in everyday life.

Chapter 4, 'Discipline and Moralism of Our Health', looks at the history of health moralism discourses and how they still pervasively circulate today via neoliberal and digital societies' advocation of digital health tools for individual self-care. I examine how self-trackers struggle to regulate their rest and legitimate inactivity, as well as perform invisible illness on social media. Shame plays a dominant role in how these individuals feel about their health management when optimal 'body image' is not upheld on social media or they are unable to maintain being a 'healthy role model'. This chapter concludes by illustrating the many burdens and challenges of everyday self-tracking and social media health performativity.

Chapter 5, 'Health "Disciples": Technology "Addiction" and Embodiment', examines the compulsive behaviours and practices of committing to healthism and performing the digital health self online via self-tracking tools and social media in everyday life. This pledge to healthism, whether conscious or not (it is often not), situates these neoliberally confirming self-managers of health optimisation, pressured and coerced by the devices and social media communities' feedback or lack thereof, into becoming micro-influencers of the digital health self. These tools of temptation are hard to resist due to the behavioural 'addictions' exacerbated by the choice architecture of the attention economy within these platforms. Lastly, this chapter discusses attempts to detox from this discipline and commitment towards healthism, as users navigate their co-evolving relationship with these technologies over time.

Chapter 6, 'Sharing "Healthiness"', looks at the broader motivations of sharing and performing the digital health self on social media in everyday life. Pressures for continuity and regular posting become a heavy consideration for self-trackers. Due to this cyclical relationship between posting and attempting to improve health and wellness, the body and diets become moulded to the aesthetics of social media and life-stylisations of health representation for these users. This chapter analyses changing social media etiquettes over time and sharing practices over time (TMI anyone?) and how problematically these etiquettes still conform to logics of gendered, idealised and sexualised bodies to gain attention and visibility under digital capitalism.

Finally, Chapter 7, 'Future Directions for the Digital Health Self', draws together our analyses in the preceding six chapters culminating in a thorough definition of the digital health self in everyday life today. I explore some of the many impacts the COVID-19 pandemic has had on our conceptualisations and management of health. Picking up from multiple assertions made in this introductory chapter, I explore stigmatisations of COVID-19, the moralism of health, surveillance and digital capitalism and what these powerful intersections mean for future health practices and research directions, as well as the broader implications for individuals, for public health and for the increasing commodifications of our bodies via digital technologies.

2

Understanding Our Bodies through Datafication

The wide adoption of self-tracking technologies by users to manage health, as well as the increasing efficacy of digital and surveillance capitalism to mine, monetise, make inferences and repurpose personal data for health profiling and targeted advertising, has led to an everyday 'datafication of health' (Ruckenstein and Schüll, 2017): the collective tools, technologies and processes used to turn many aspects of our lifestyle and health into data and new forms of value exchange. This chapter examines these conceptual and practical shifts towards the datafication of health that self-tracking technologies and social media have brought about through a theoretical and empirical analytical approach, drawing on data from interviews, reflexive diaries and online content. Through different technological, practical and economic shifts, from the self-quantification movement to consumer self-tracking to the increasing everyday datafication of health and digital phenotyping, this chapter traces how data collection, mining and sharing have become an integral part of health management and self-care for users, citizens and patients under digital capitalism. Through behavioural economic theories of choice architecture and nudge theory (Thaler and Sunstein, 2009) the chapter argues for the need to pay ethical attention to the persuasive and coercive design within self-tracking and digital health technologies. It analyses the impact of health gamification (Whitson, 2015) and what it means when we understand our health, body, and identity through data, current debates in new materialism (Barad, 2007, 2014; Braidotti, 2018; Lupton, 2019) and the political economy of the datafication of health (Moore, 2018). The chapter concludes by considering the ongoing and long-term assemblage of humans with the reductive patterns of datafication and how these processes can promote the regulation and agential (re)organisation of bodily experience of the digital health self through everyday reductive processes of datafication.

From self-quantification to self-tracking

To understand the practices and implications of datafication upon health management, I must start by analysing its relationship to self-quantification. Self-quantification is the reliance upon science and the technological extensions and affordances of scientific sensors in the monitoring of the self and individual health (Wolf, 2010). Users of the 'quantified self' (QS) movement monitor, through consumer devices, everything that can be put into data to 'improve' and 'optimize' individual health. Gary Wolf, co-founder (with Kevin Kelly) of the movement, has called it 'self-knowledge through numbers' (Wolf, 2010). The QS movement came from a California-based laboratory, which now has an international collaboration of users and makers of self-training tools (Swan, 2009). Swan (2013: 86) understands self-quantification as 'contemporary formalizations belonging to the general progression in human history of using measurement, science, and technology to bring order, understanding, manipulation, and control to the natural world, including the human body'. The QS movement, or rather its practices of capturing data, can be broadly described as 'self-tracking': the process of tracking aspects of our bodies and our minds, which promotes 'an exploratory worldview in which the key goal is learning through the process of data collection and interpretation' (Fajans, 2013: np). This perspective takes a particularly techno-utopian angle, similar to that of Nafus and Sherman (2014), who suggest that self-quantification could be considered as an alternative to big data practices since self-management could be considered emancipatory when compared to the perspective of wider state surveillance. It is also important to recognise that the QS movement (Wolf, 2010) is a key demonstration of neoliberal self-management and self-surveillance practices, which, like the earlier 1980s discourse advocated by Thatcher's government, prioritise individual choice as a mechanism for the self-improvement of health.

Digital health practices and the affordances of self-tracking devices and social media have dimensions of both self-surveillance and wider surveillance, as I shall explore more in Chapter 3, 'Surveillance Cultures of the Digital Health Self'. These arguments are relevant for our analysis into the datafication of health as tools for and techniques of bodily monitoring and, arguably, control. For example, Robins and Webster (1999: 180) argue that such types of 'social control [have become] more pervasive, more invasive, more total, but also more routine, mundane and inescapable'. Therefore, such self-surveillance may, in fact, be normalised, even 'desired', as a way of proving individual responsibility within neoliberal advocated citizenship practices and behaviours: 'these surveillant assemblages are ideally configured voluntarily, as laypeople judge their participation in self-surveillance as being in their own best interests' (Lupton, 2013b: 12). Self-tracking, therefore, ensures that the body and health are 'being subjected to regimes of knowledge production and data-driven modes of bio-power' (Ajana, 2017: 2). These regimes of bio-power and neoliberal judgement dictate which are and which are not healthy, productive and self-bettering behaviours subsumed through discourses of competition and comparison (Cederstrom and Spicer, 2015; Davies, 2016). Let us now explore the relationship between self-quantification, self-tracking and the datafication of health.

As Chapter 1 argued, both the quantitative tracking and qualitative representations of health, fitness, diet and lifestyle can be conceived as practices of self-tracking in the digital society of today. Swan (2012a) identifies three layers to self-tracking technologies: firstly, input via sensors and devices; secondly, analysis via algorithms and signal processing; and lastly, services via visualisation, storage, and feedback. This book proposes a fourth aspect: the way users may use their data and visualisations to self-represent certain 'health' identities. It is through these self-representations that comparisons between 'healthy' bodies and lifestyles can be made; in turn, competition can also act as a motivator for self-trackers:

> The great appeal of the competition, from the neoliberal perspective, is that it enables activity to be rationalised and quantified, but in ways that purport to maintain uncertainty of outcome. The promise of competition is to provide a form of socio-economic objectivity that is empirically and mathematically knowable but still possessed of its own internal dynamism and vitality. (Davies, 2015: 41–42)

This book analyses user engagement with these practices of 'knowing thyself' (Wolf and Kelly, 2007), through self-quantification and self-tracking technologies, in how they produce knowledge and different understandings of the body through self-representations on social media. This chapter then examines the problematic aspects of identifying with and understanding one's own body through such data capture and 'this growing trend of self-quantification and data-driven modes of health monitoring, particularly with regard to issues of privacy and data ownership as well as the marked shifts in healthcare responsibilities' (Ajana, 2017: 2). This may worryingly become embodied by the users themselves, for if 'health' becomes situated as best managed through these commercially mined self-tracking technologies, privacy is repackaged as in opposition to the 'collective' and 'public good', which is framed as making populations 'healthier' through data mining (Ajana, 2017: 2). This philanthropic data discourse, which in recent years has attempted to legitimate data mining and privacy invasions, ensures that 'privacy is dead, and profit is king (...), any reuse of data beyond the original purpose for which it was collected is a potential threat to privacy and civil liberties' (Kirkpatrick, 2017: 11), which is not always recognised or fully understood by the users themselves. As Kelvin (1973) argues, the role of privacy becomes a nullification mechanism for advocating surveillance. Therefore, voluntary self-surveillant practices of self-trackers problematically play directly into state discourses, as well as capitalist and corporate profit strategies.

From self-tracking to the datafication of health

The quantitative and qualitative aspects of self-tracking mean that data related to and illustrative of self-tracking is concerned with how numbers, graphs and statistics, as well as photographic representations of the body, (gym) 'selfies', food or exercise equipment (yoga mats or bicycles, for example), all provide the ability to capture the messiness and multidimensional aspects of one's life in 'controllable life slices' (Ruckenstein, 2017: 6). Elliot and Urry (2010: 6) argue that individually quantifying behaviours and habits, generated via 'miniaturised mobilities', 'enable(s) people to deposit affects, moods and dispositions into techno-objects'. However, increased reliance upon self-tracking and digital health tools, as well as navigating a wealth of (mis)information online, including social media influencer culture and its lack of regulation, means that we as a society are ever more unclear about what 'healthiness' means. Moreover, individuals have become ever more reliant upon scientific experts; a by-product of the function creep of social media influencers in neoliberal and digital capitalist times means that some are qualified to share health information whereas many are not, leaving unqualified 'lifestyle influencers' circulating potentially harmful guidance and advice to unknowing audiences. The sheer abundance of data and nutritional information available further complicates 'health (mis)information', as everyone becomes an 'expert' on optimising good health. As Kristensen and Ruckenstein (2018: 12) assert: 'sensors and devices [have] become part of the processes in which the self is defined, extended, reduced, or restricted.' So, how do users, patients and citizens actually self-track, quantify and utilise digital health technologies to self-manage health? The impacts of these shifts are huge. For example, between 67 per cent and 92 per cent of teenagers report using social media for health information (fitness, sexual health and nutrition); however, many are unable to identify reliable information and often they use social media more than National Health Service, Public Health England and the Department of Health websites (Plaisme, 2020). This is a worrying and pervasive problem that will only become exacerbated in time if social media continues to evade the regulation of health-related informational and guidance content.

Surveillance cultures of the digital health self

Furthermore, digital health, self-tracking and wellness apps renegotiate the boundaries between medical and consumer products. These lifestyle choices are conceptualised and referred to as different 'styles of living, which in turn are shaped by their patterns of consumption' (Nettleton, 2013: 3). This creates ambiguities and 'challenges implicit distinctions between what is medical and what is related to personal lifestyle choices within current regulatory systems' (Lucievo and Prainsack, 2015: 1). The participatory elements of web 2.0–3.0 digital society ensure we can increasingly collect larger amounts of data on many aspects of our bodies; tracking geo-location, emotion and physical function is now an everyday normative practice through many application-based tracking services such as My Fitness Pal and Nike Run Club and tracking sensors such as Fitbit, Strava, Garmin or Apple Watch. However, they are interestingly framed within policy and the media as having the capacity to transform behaviour and encourage 'healthy' lifestyles. Such technologies are often celebrated as 'revolutionising' healthcare and promise to optimise individual health through reflexive self-regulating practices The gaze of medical professionals, a once status-infused level of expertise, ensured that self-monitoring of bodily functions and self-diagnosis were once impossible for the patient or citizen; however, now anyone with access to digital health or self-tracking technologies can access diagnostic information as well as have the ability to monitor one's own health or ailments via these technologies (Lupton, 2012a). Today, the wider public has the oppportunity to frequently monitor and 'traverse between what is inside and outside the body' (Nafus and Sherman, 2014: 6). To some extent, citizens and laypeople can now adopt a medical gaze.

Patients and consumers using these platforms to manage their health 'frequently engage with medicine in a manner that integrates diagnosis, treatment, and research' (Prainsack, 2013: 112). Although we could all be affected by illness or disease that we could not have protected ourselves from, the neoliberal individualisation discourse places responsibility in the hands of the sufferer: 'If (…) people suffer from illnesses as a result of allegedly deliberate actions or actions against better knowledge, then they are to be taken to be accountable and indeed responsible for their condition' (Buyx and Prainsack, 2012: 81). These arguments advocate individual health responsibilisation as the rhetoric to support digital health applications and self-tracking; '[O]ur personal understanding of who we are connected within the sense of reorganising similarity in a relevant respect – shapes our judgements of what situations people should be held accountable for' (Buyx and Prainsack, 2012: 81). Digital health technology, however, does attempt to fill this void with discourses of health management and 'evidence-based optimism' (Buyx and Prainsack, 2012: 81), through health 'optimisation'. Discussions around who is responsible for poor health 'distract the attention of policymakers from addressing the underlying and hugely important social determinants of health' (Buyx and Prainsack, 2012: 82). In the context of risk society (Beck, 1992: 3) the risk is contextual to what we examine and look at: 'it can be seen as a concept created to allow the quantification of circumstances and situations that do not really lend themselves to quantification'. Different perspectives on these individual and political practices stem from, at one end, seeing this self-monitoring as increasing control and enabling autonomy in one's health management (Beato, 2012). At the other, more critical, end of the analysis, Heyes (2006: 145) considers how individuals may struggle to engage with (digital) health practices without becoming 'the projected unified subject of its regime'. Beato (2012) and Heyes (2006) take an arguably limited view, which does not take into consideration self-governance as an extension of neoliberal controlling rationalities and the market priorities of data and surveillance capitalism underpinning social media and consumer digital health platforms.

From the datafication of health to digital phenotyping

Datafication refers to the conversion of qualitative aspects of life into quantifiable data (Mayer-Schönberger and Cukier, 2013). In the context of health, this can be understood as the process by which qualitative aspects of life are recorded as quantifiable data and made analysable in terms of health. The ability to make inferences about health from data and the ability to repurpose data about health are two defining features of the datafication of health, affording those with control over or access to data extensive possibilities to influence people's lives and health (Ada Lovelace Institute, 2020). For example, if a user is tracking their calories using My Fitness Pal to monitor their calorie intake, they input and scan each item that is consumed throughout their day; drink, food and physical activity, such as energy expenditure, are also inputted to calculate how many calories that user has consumed, burnt off from exercise and absorbed that day. On the one hand, this is useful to self-trackers to monitor aspects of their health (whatever is being tracked, nutrition, diet or exercise). However, the benefits of consuming x number of calories per day (for a man or woman) is defined not by the nutritional content of the calories, such as highly nutritious (a banana) versus junk foods or foods high in salt, fat or sugar (biscuit) content, but by the number of calories they consumed. The user may consume a biscuit or a banana with the same number of calories, but each has varying and different nutritional qualities (or lack thereof) and impacts upon an individual's energy levels and source of fuel for the human body. Therefore, consuming 2000 calories from junk foods on the device might appear 'healthy' as daily calorie goals are met, but nutrition and health goals are not. Therefore, this 'datafication of health' (Ruckenstein and Schull, 2017: 262) also affects health qualitatively as this shifts definitions and practices of what 'healthy' is by generating an ongoing need to consider what a 'healthy' relationship between people and their data looks like (Ada Lovelace Institute, 2020). It is like placing a filter over a full body selfie in tight gym clothes to make your body look leaner. Your body might look healthier and more 'attractive' through the visual register of sexualised, slim objectifications of what we deem 'Insta-worthy' healthy bodies online, but the filter is not an arbiter of truth but a barrier to authenticity. The fact that a fit and healthy user even considers using a filter to alter their form highlights the many problems that surround social media representation of healthy and fit bodies, alongside the related reductive and oversimplified portrayal of 'health' through datafication.

The amount of data about health that can be collected from everyday activity has grown rapidly in recent years; aside from voluntary self-tracking from digital health tools, advertisers are predicting and marketing health, wellbeing and fitness products to us recommended by algorithms predicting our next health-related purchase interest. A way to understand the pervasiveness of this datafication of health in everyday life is through the concept of 'digital phenotyping' (Jain et al, 2015), a term developed in 2015, which is 'the moment-by-moment quantification of the individual-level phenotype in situ using data from personal digital devices' (Ada Lovelace Institute, 2020: 9). This means our personal data can be analysed to infer our personal health status, for example, by social media analytics companies rather than traditional healthcare settings such as a GP surgery or hospital (Ada Lovelace Institute, 2020). Similarly, the data can be repurposed and used for purposes unrelated or not directly related to healthcare, such as risk assessments for insurance premiums (Ada Lovelace Institute, 2020). What this means is that a wealth and variety of public and private actors, such as governments, healthcare systems, the tech industry, employers and insurers, can now have access to, make inferences from and repurpose our health and personal data. Our digital traces across networked platforms can then be used to generate insights and predictions about our health, blurring the 'perceived boundaries of the body, meaning it is possible to make algorithmically driven inferences about health based on disembodied data about people' (Ada Lovelace Institute, 2020: 8). While we can to an extent consider platforms as a medium to represent and shape public health, privacy is also dependent on the user's proficiency and expertise with the website or application, as well as the choice architecture, design and technological restrictions of the platform. Furthermore, the varying process of mediation, which shapes self-representations, is contextual and dependent on the user's ability to manage the 'public-ness' of the content within privacy settings. Therefore, the proliferation of the datafication of health, and COVID-19 as the first pandemic of the algorithmic age (Ada Lovelace Institute, 2020), raises many ethical and practical concerns about privacy and surveillance by the state, tech companies and other citizens (peer surveillance) (Kent, 2020), as the boundaries of what is or is not data about health are no longer clear (Ada Lovelace Institute, 2020).

> By converting aspects of people's lives into quantifiable data, technologies shape the conscious and unconscious choices people make about their health. This creates a 'symbiotic agency' where technologies mediate human experience and affect human agency, while human agency simultaneously shapes the uses of these technologies. (Lupton, 2017: 8)

The transformation of social action into online quantified data, which has ultimately allowed for real-time tracking and predictive analysis, has now become a legitimate means to access, understand and monitor people's behaviour and, in turn, is identifying new social behaviour and cultural norms given the vast amounts of social and cultural practices that have now been datafied. With the capability to track and monitor expanding aspects of our bodies, 'increasingly, the market sees you from within, measuring your body and emotional states, and watching you as you move around' (Fourcade and Healy, 2017: 23). There are considerable benefits to the datafication of health. Not only can individuals be better informed about their health but advances in data analytics also lay the foundations for artificial intelligence solutions in diagnosis, personalisation and prevention in medicine. However, datafication raises significant concerns too. It makes individuals' health status available to a broad array of actors outside recognised medical and clinical settings, giving those with the appropriate digital tools an increased ability to know about, and engage with, people's health through their data (Ada Lovelace Institute, 2020). Datafication also produces increasingly comprehensive renderings of health, creating the potential conditions for disempowerment for individuals, and opportunities to monitor and influence people in ways never seen before. In other words, our everyday digital traces are mined and profiled to the extent that it is now arguable that 'all data is health data' (Warzel, 2019).

The choice architecture of coercive self-tracking technologies

The assumption made, as well as the narrative marketed, by the tech industry, and often depicted by the press and news media, is that datafication and more monitoring and tracking of personal behaviour and activity will yield helpful insights for health management and illness prevention for public health. Whilst to some extent this might be true, what also needs attention within conversations around the datafication of health is the choice architecture of the digital health devices and self-tracking apps that consumers and patients use to monitor, 'improve' and 'optimise' their health, fitness and diet. The current figures for consumer digital health technology valued globally highlight the cause for concern. In 2022, the market value for consumer (only) digital health tech was $334 billion, predicted to grow to a global market value of $657 billion by 2025 (Statistica, 2021). It is fair to say this is a highly lucrative, widely adopted, and thus pervasively integrated market. Therefore, the motivation behind the design and choice architecture of digital health applications in influencing user behaviours demands further investigation and regulation. Beato (2012) describes the embodiment of decision-making within a technological device as 'choice architecture'. A choice architect holds the responsibility for organising specific contexts and environments in which people, in this case users and consumers, make decisions (Thaler and Sunstein, 2009: 3). This strategy evolves from behavioural economics and is proposed by Richard Thaler and Cass Sunstein (2009) as the best way to help people make decisions; as they argue, a

> false assumption is that almost all people, almost all of the time, make choices that are in their best interest or at the very least are better than the choices that would be made by someone else. We claim that this assumption is false—indeed, obviously false. In fact, we do not think that anyone believes it on reflection. (Thaler and Sunstein, 2009: 6)

Thaler and Sunstein argue in their seminal book *Nudge* (2009) that the choice architect then becomes best placed to direct and shape decision-making and outcomes for consumers. I do not agree, and my research findings also demonstrate otherwise. The motive and incentive of the choice architect must be considered, particularly in the context of the business models of surveillance and digital capitalism that underpin our current digital society and the use of digital health and self-tracking devices, tools and platforms. Choice architecture as a method of behavioural economics, has been met with some scepticism and reflects a potential commitment to actively bias people in ways that could easily be seen as persuasive or coercive. For example, as a quick aside, when analysing self-representations online it is important to recognise that platform developers and associated institutions algorithmically construct who sees what, who the audience is and which content will be available to them through the choice architecture of the platform. Therefore, 'the question of whether platforms for self-representation are publicly funded or profit-driven for example, and crucially, to whom they are accountable, are key aspects of the process of institutional mediation shaping any self-representation that takes place' (Thumin, 2012: 39). One key example of this is was during COVID-19, when the UK Conservative government paid influencers to promote 'track and trace' on their Instagram profiles (BBC News, 2020): '7 million people have been reached', said a spokesman for the government, 'This is just one part of a wider campaign utilising TV, radio, social, print and other advertisements to ensure the public has the information it needs.' Shaughna Phillips, who has 1.5 million followers on Instagram, posted on 17 August 2020 that she wanted to remind her audience 'about the importance of coronavirus testing'. She stated that being tested was 'totally free, quick and is vital to stop the spread of coronavirus'. It is worth noting that influencers with over a million followers on Instagram can earn up to $20,000 (£14,980) per post they make on behalf of advertisers and that this was paid using public funds for public health messaging without UK citizens' knowledge (BBC News, 2020). The big question is, is this ethical? It certainly raises challenges to the contentious argument to how public health messaging is and should be delivered in the current digital society.

Gamification and 'nudging' the digital health self

The advocating of digital health tools from tech giants, and within public health promotional policy, particularly during COVID-19, is deserving of urgent analysis. Identifying digital health technologies as a powerful marketing tool within new health promotion practices draws attention to the ethical implications of the platform's choice architecture, especially in recommending their use to consumers. Therefore, choice architecture and regulatory design tools of these applications and devices may 'nudge' and prompt users to make certain 'health' choices (such as lower calorie consumption) and to undertake certain health behaviours (such as exercising or running further).

> A nudge (…) is any aspect of the choice architecture that alters people's behavior in a predictable way without forbidding any options or significantly changing their economic incentives. (Thaler and Sunstein, 2009: 6)

If our behaviour changes as a direct result of being 'nudged' by a design driver, in response to wider socio-cultural and political priorities and pressures, this could have enormous ethical implications in terms of the motivations behind such designs. Nudging as a concept and practice has also been increasingly used in public health interventions in western societies with the goal to produce behaviour change and push healthier lifestyle changes (Lederer et al, 2020). As an intervention it is used to prompt behaviours that may result in health improvements in populations (Marteau et al, 2011; Vallgårda, 2012; Saghai, 2013). A potentially dangerous aspect of 'nudging' within these applications is that it is leading the self-tracker to become reliant on the device for health management and thus potentially ignore or disregard human instinct. Following the 'nudge' from a health or fitness device, like a calorie counter or running app, might prompt the user to consume less calories (and get the nutrition they need), or encourage a runner to force themselves out when they have an injury or perhaps their energy is depleted for any variety of reasons. Alarmingly, 'nudging' as a practice contributes to the discourse of self-quantification being reflective of health improvement, whereby human activity, capacity and behaviours become reduced to numbers, to a human version of computing, which doesn't take into consideration all human senses and attributes. Being continually notified and 'nudged' by the app of the time and distance left to go on a running app can remind the user of the challenges ahead, which may not be achieved and thus can cause anxiety for the user.

Purpura et al (2011) argue that the functions of these applications must be recognised as powerful regulatory tools that arguably coerce users to undertake certain actions that cannot be individually tailored to each user and may therefore inflict damaging physical pressure upon the body as well as additional psychological pressure on the minds of the users. App developers would argue that these socio-technological 'nudges' motivate the user. However, this sometimes fails, as this 'nudge' is interpreted as controlling and at times demotivating. This challenges dominant discourses around these consumer products, which stipulate that self-tracking devices support and enable 'healthier' decisions and 'healthier' bodies. The body is not a machine and cannot be technologically 'controlled', managed or 'optimised' in this way. Quigley (2013: 588) expands on this, by asserting that device 'nudges' 'can be conceived as part of an expanding arsenal of health-affecting regulatory tools (…) used by government [and commerce] and addresses some concerns which have been expressed regarding behavioural research-driven regulation and policy'. This is a hugely important and potentially problematic aspect of such digital health and self-tracking devices that needs addressing. As mentioned earlier, if users' behaviour change as a result of 'nudges' by a design driver, in response to wider socio-cultural and political priorities and pressures, this could have considerable ethical implications in terms of the motivations behind such designs, as demonstrated by Lou's entries here:

> NRC [Nike Running Club] meant I didn't cut my run short when it felt hard/when I thought I was on my planned route, but had I not checked I wouldn't have run the full distance I needed to. (Lou, diary entry, 29, F)

> I also set NRC today to my goal distance. I did this as it was a new feature and seemed quite interesting. I didn't actually realise how motivating it was to have it count down how much further, which was really helpful. (Lou, diary entry, 29, F)

While a 'nudge' might be motivating, it is important to recognise that these devices cannot take into consideration individual emotional wellbeing, physical stress or trauma within the data capture. The increased self-knowledge gained through these applications encourages increased individual reflexivity, which is 'embedded within particular normative discursive framings of choice' (Adams and Raisborough, 2008: 1171). Therefore, self-surveillance becomes an individualised pressure cycle of standardised meritocracy, further enhancing the increased need for self-knowledge (Langwieser and Kirig, 2010), Furthermore, as Moore (2017: np) argues, 'Nudge as a method has been met with some scepticism and reflects a commitment to actively bias people in ways that could easily be seen as "creepy".' Alongside work and lifestyle-influencing health decisions, these digital mediations of individual health practices (whether shared or monitored personally) contribute to anxieties related to a perceived lack of self-discipline, poor body image and other problematic aspects of self-tracking such as invasive (self-) surveillance and invasions of personal privacy.

'Health gamification' is enabled by digital health technologies and applications that promise to make our everyday lives more like a game. Gamification can be understood as incorporating game elements into a non-game context (Whitson, 2013). These mobile, wearable devices and applications were frequently considered a 'new toy' by the users, demonstrating how both the technologies and their usage align themselves with a gamification of health. With self-tracking technologies, this is enabled on applications through badges, points, graphs and leader boards, as well as through non-gaming activities such as calorie counting, running, cycling and sleep tracking. Therefore, similar to the knowledge by numbers and knowledge by data discourses that surround both self-tracking and self-quantification, health gamification operates through an instrumentalisation of play and play by numbers:

> 'I had a ridiculous run where I had 16 or 18 miles and actually that's always a bit soul destroying at that sort of distance because even when you've run really far you've still got really far to go, and I think the flipside of that [you think] "are you kidding me, I've still got 10 miles to go". I just want to lay down in this bush and stay here for a couple of hours. I think I turned it off then because I was just like "I don't need to hear that". I just need to know that I've done the distance and check in on myself.' (Lou, final interview, 29, F)

In this case, the app reminding the participant of the time left to run was far from encouraging but was rather demotivating and soul deflating. Therefore, the application can be seen as capable of limiting or extending human capabilities depending upon the goals provided by the device. This form of persuasive computing encourages a scientific rationalisation of everyday life. Regardless of personal circumstances or external factors, it 'values quantification and rationality at the cost of situational, hard-to-measure factors and sees scientific measurement as obviating personal experience'

(Purpura et al, 2011: 6). As discussed earlier, this discourse argues that self-quantification reduces human activity and behaviours to numbers, to a human version of computing, which doesn't take into consideration all human senses and attributes. Furthermore, the optimisation of the self-improvement cycle never ends and holds as much weight (in terms of acknowledging personal fitness development) for the individual as the actual physical improvement, as this user acknowledged:

> 'There was a time when I would've looked at me now and been well happy with it but now I think I look at a lot of pictures of people online and even though I know they're photo-shopped I feel like I need to look like that, I need abs like that, I need my arms to look like that.' (Sophie, final interview, 31, F)

Fitness development and muscle 'gains' are often goals that are never achieved or fully reached, for these health-focused individuals, much like the health gamification on the devices, these practices never end within self-monitoring and peer surveillance cultures. In turn, this could damage self-esteem through feelings of failure or inadequacy when comparing ourselves to others. As Thacker (2003: 56) describes in his theory of cultural attitudes towards the body and bio-media more broadly: 'our culture wants to render the body immediate, while also multiplying our capacity to technically control the body.' The immediacy of the body is enabled for Lou in the aforementioned quote through the regulatory design 'nudges' reminding her of the distance to go. Treating bodies as data moves life 'beyond the body-as-organism; these biotechnologies (...) make it possible to treat life capacities or affectivity as a matter of "non-organic-life", the latter referring to a conception of bodily matter or matter generally, where the capacity for self-organisation is understood to be immanent to matter' (Clough, 2010: 1–2). However, all human activity – physical, mental or emotional – cannot be fully confined within self-tracking devices and platforms, limiting our definition of what needs scientific grounding and explanation. These devices are not just about enlightenment through data but about information produced to change users' behaviours.

Users explained how this reminded them to 'be healthier', in whatever way that was subjectively interpreted, clearly demonstrating how the consumer apps, devices and social media that promote 'healthier' activities nudge and advocate their use, which in turn pushes users' behaviours to respond.

> We are capturing everything, so our conclusions are not relevant to every person or to every situation. So how do you summarise and symbolise without oversimplification and distortion? (Duffy, 2014: np)

Visualising our data through these interfaces could similarly be considered problematic, since through this semiotic layer of representation the data story is 'revealed' but also represented in an arguably sensationalist way (Ruckenstein, 2017). Examples of participants' self-tracked running data are shown in Figures 2.1 and 2.2. In the sense that the quantified self and self-tracking movement is concerned with self-awareness by numbers or data (Wolf, 2010), a representation of data is similarly created either through a new medium or reproduction; a new visualisation of data to make it meaningful. So, although medics use diagnostic technologies, which produce health data, the difference here is that non-medical or 'laypeople' attempt to understand their bodies through sensationalised visual representations of data from digital health devices. Their perceptions of the digitised reproduction of bodily monitoring and biometrics may influence how this information is internalised and then acted upon by the self-tracker.

Figure 2.1: Example of participant self-tracking data

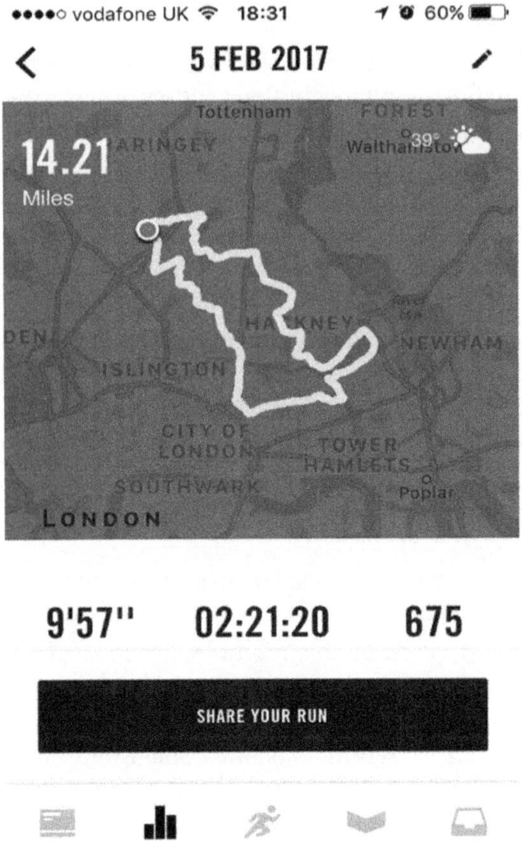

Figure 2.2: Example of participant running data

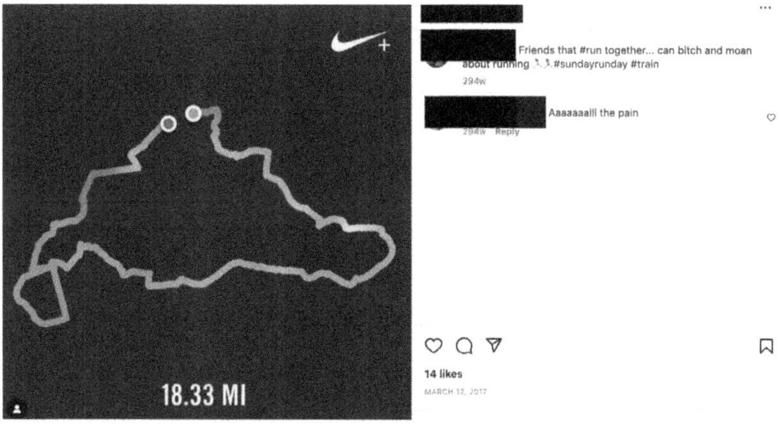
18.33 MI
Friends that #run together... can bitch and moan
#sundayrunday #train
294w
Aaaaaaalll the pain
14 likes
MARCH 12, 2017

Therefore, health 'gamification' can be understood as a form of health strategisation, whereby users of self-tracking technologies use gaming and play to self-survey health behaviours and outcomes and work towards rewards systems such as badges, medals or leader boards on the applications themselves. The following diary entry by Lou shows how improving upon time and distance became a key demonstration of self-maintenance through individual regulation and self-improvement. This corroborates the mediation and processes of persuasive or coercive computing (Purpura et al, 2011) about digital health devices and practices and governance of the (emotional) self (Foucault, 1979a; Rose, 1999). This focus to maximise our happiness through scrutiny over and management of health, like with those fixated upon wellness-seeking, constructs a pervasive practice that 'slowly edges out the rest of the world, what is left is the repetitive pulsation of the body' (Cederstrom and Spicer, 2015: 91). In this case the body adheres to technological sensors; it is moved and shaped in adherence to the design in motivation to achieve optimal goals and individual perceptions of success.

> The marathon was the main goal. I was probably more in tune with pace due to it being more visible (on my wrist). Which was motivating. (Lou, diary entry, 29, F)

We escape into games, but we also exercise our 'hyper rationalised mind into managing an actuarial risk' (Whitson, 2013: np). In this regard, we understand health as something that needs to be managed and maintained, through the careful consideration of risk, ill health, disease and ultimately death. As Fotopoulou and O'Riordan (2016: 66) highlight, these 'commercial tracking devices are promoted as leisure and fitness devices [which] places them in the category of knowledge for prevention, which is also experiential and personal'. The game we are playing through self-tracking devices and platforms is about our human bodies and, most importantly, our human capabilities. Health gamification through nudges, therefore, is a game of self-governance created through the feedback loops held within these devices, a management and enactment of self-governance and control, to manage ongoing and everyday health risks.

Quantifying narratives of the digital healthy self

Aside from what, where and why self-trackers were sharing their content, one of the first interview questions asked in this research was: 'What does the word health mean to you?' Given that the participants were recruited based on their sharing health-related content on Facebook and Instagram, interestingly most were confused by this question and struggled to identify what the significance of 'health' was for them. This highlighted the many conceptualisations, wide ambiguity and varied understandings of what 'health' meant to self-trackers whose lifestyles centred around attempts to maintain 'good health'. During the interviews, the users were often prompted by being asked: 'What is healthy?' A wide range of responses were received, ranging from quantified 'health' to physical ability and mental wellbeing. For Fet, a keen cyclist who tracked his daily work commute, 'health' was quantifiable through metrics and being 'healthy' was determined by his body weight:

> 'Mine is a number, and my number is 65 kg, and if I'm above 65 kg I consider myself as "unhealthy". For me I could be 66 kg or I could be 80 kg. There's no difference: as long as I go above that benchmark. I know I'm eating well, yeah. I have the odd kebab or Chinese on the weekend but in general during the week I eat well. I would consider myself a healthy eater. When it comes to health overall (…) if I'm above 65 kg, which I've set myself, I don't know why or how, I think mainly because that's my weight roughly, for the past ten years because I haven't really changed in terms of my weight, so if I go above that mark by 1 kg or 10 kg I'm unhealthy.' (Fet, first interview, 30, M)

Fet 'set' and determined his 'health' by numerical weight. His reasoning was interestingly unclear to him. However, the use of numbers to determine his 'healthiness' was becaue of the consistency of being approximately a certain weight over a ten-year period. Interestingly, his rationale for determining whether he was 'unhealthy' or not was related to being above this 'set' weight of 65 kg, regardless of the relative increase in metrics. For example, being 75 kg or 100 kg was not a determinant of degrees of 'un-healthiness'. Quite simply, for Fet, weighing over 65 kg had a causal relationship with being 'unhealthy'. Therefore, the physical deterioration of health was understood through numerical weight gain, regardless of other mental or physical factors such as illness, disease, lack of nutrition or exercise (in his case, cycling). Fet's perspective resonated with Purpura et al's (2011: 6) argument concerning the recognition of the 'idea that sensors accurately measure attributes that directly translate to health; that health can be measured [works] in a purely reductive way'. For Fet, being healthy was being his goal weight. Quantifying his health in this way arguably meant that Fet did not have to take into consideration the self-regulation of many other lifestyle factors that could impact on 'healthiness' (such as exercise). By relying on this simplified quantification system, Fet understood his health through numbers in line with the discourse advocated by the self-quantification community, supporting 'self-knowledge by numbers' (Wolf and Kelly, 2010). These reductive approaches to understanding and managing health reflect how the users' interpretations of what determines 'good health' or 'ill health' are strongly encoded by their own technological, medical and cultural assumptions (Roach, 2017), which create categories of importance. Several questions can therefore be asked: What data do we collect and why should we identify 'healthiness'? How does this reflect cultural, technological and medical assumptions and discourses concerning what is 'healthy' or 'unhealthy'?

Lucivero and Prainsack (2015: 2) argue that 'new technologies challenge our symbolic order, that is, the grid of concepts that are used in a certain society to order and categorise reality'. In the context of digital health and self-tracking technologies, the distinctions between the physical body, data and the mind are renegotiated and shift our normative definitions and understandings of what we consider a 'body' and a 'person' (Lucivero and Tamburrini, 2007). Therefore, if I take a new materialist perspective, this 'allows for the conceptualisation of the travelling of the fluxes of matter and mind, body and soul, nature and culture' (Dolphijn, 2010: 2), which attends to enabling the examination into the shifts and definition of what we deem to be 'healthy' individuals, and patients as sufferers of ill health, in whichever capacity it is determined or captured. Felton (2014) argues that stories are how our human brain makes sense of our environments. For biological data to be meaningful it has to become more than simply biological: 'now that data is this elemental part of our lives, we have to translate it into stories in order to make it meaningful or operational for us' (Felton, 2014: np). What Felton (2014) means is that data by itself cannot be enough to become meaningful or relevant; we have to create narratives through data, whether it be at a large societal scale, for example socio-epidemiological considerations, or at an individualised level as a representation of our identity and self. Perhaps from here, we can understand the motivations behind the QS movement and the uptake of consumer self-tracking practices more broadly. As Moore and Robinson (2016: 2775) argue, the assumptions driving the quantified self (in the workplace) and arguably shifts towards self-tracking more broadly sit on an 'ontological premise of Cartesian dualism with mind dominant over body'. QS movement founder Gary Wolf (2010: np) considers the motivations behind the QS movement, and arguably self-tracking, as 'self-awareness through data'. Self-awareness, however, is a subjective and ironically unquantifiable term. How can one determine if they are fully self-aware through a device or machine when the unquantifiable becomes disregarded and health is reduced in this oversimplified way? As Thacker (2003: 48) expands: 'It is not just the medium [that] is the message, but that biology is the new medium: the medium is a message and that message is a molecule.' Therefore, bio-media assumes that human bodies 'are informed by a single assumption: that there exists some fundamental equivalency between genetic "codes" and computer "codes", or between the biological and informatic domains, such that they can be rendered interchangeable in terms of materials and functions' (Thacker, 2003: 52). In other words, bio-media cannot always consider the non-sequential and somatic nature of ill health and disease. In doing so, we disregard the elements that we cannot quantify or neatly capture, in turn increasingly limiting our understanding of life itself and, within it, pathologies and 'health'. Creating narratives from our data helps makes our self-tracking data relatable, personal and humanised.

'Likes' as currency

Perceiving the online community as an audience who participated through feedback on posts was a key motivator for users to track and share their health and fitness practices on social media. Speaking to, for and with the audience ensured that discussion and recognition of health improvement and fitness development became collaborative through the participation of sharers and their communities. This personal gratification and participation are quantified through feedback. On Facebook and Instagram, this comes in the form of 'likes' and written support for posts.

> 'The likes, that's your currency.' (Jennie, first interview, 40, F)

The currency of quantifying 'liking', as with the currency of self-tracking data acquisition and self-representational tools, provided the users with a sense of personal accomplishment, reflecting Moore and Robinson's (2016: 2778) argument that 'capitalism seeks to rationalise the process of cultural production through expanded quantification'. Acquiring more 'likes' meant increasing regular posting, regardless of the amount of time and effort spent. More posting made the users feel healthier, as this became representative of their 'digital health self', even if idealised. Interestingly, if this was not achieved once content was shared, technology was often blamed.

> 'If I only got one like on a picture I'd be like "is something not working?", I know it's really shallow.' (Sophie, first interview, 31, F)

> Likes on photo were motivational. Motivation on sharing this run – it was really hard work today. Expected as I was tired, but it was also very grey and cold, and I got lost. Was in pain and exhausted so this was the first time that the likes have been a bit of a motivational boost – like a social media pat on the back of sorts. (Lou, diary entry, 29, F)

> The comments from my friends definitely encouraged me to do this more often as I appeared to look healthy to them and in myself, I felt awesome too. (Tim, diary entry, 34, M)

Receiving 'likes' is social media's way of providing users with a virtual 'pat on the back', motivating further 'healthy' behaviours. In turn, the acquisition of 'likes' form a currency related to social and health status, as well as reputation management. As van Dijck (2013a: 202) explains: '"liking" has turned into a provoked automated gesture that yields precious information about people's desires and predilections.' Having a reputation as a 'healthy' and fit person offers a quantifiable status through audience or community surveillance and feedback in the form of 'likes'. The online community and network become a 'quantifiable metric for social status (…) The ability to attract and command attention becomes a status symbol' (Marwick and boyd, 2010: 12). The supportive aspect and the recognition that people are observing your activity and 'liking' certain behaviours contribute to a wider sense of self and belonging within one's health community of interest. This ensures that the sharer knows the community deems them 'fit'. In turn, they embody this health identity and thus their management of 'healthy' reputation remains intact.

Chapter 6, 'Sharing "Healthiness"', will examine in more detail this construction of an idealised healthy online self. For this chapter, however, the role of 'likes' is the most noteworthy phenomenon. The participants frequently spoke about the amount of time spent curating posts to ensure 'enough' likes were received. However, a recurrent theme was that the number of 'likes' received reduced their paranoia of being perceived in the 'wrong' way. Such bad perceptions were identified as 'oversharing', being narcissistic or being an 'obsessive health freak'. However, oversharing was deemed worse than not sharing 'healthy' behaviours, for fear of being judged and perceived negatively by the community. How many 'likes' is 'enough' was individually determined by the users, crucially in line with their own sense of self-esteem whilst simultaneously being compared to previous posts. If the users were feeling 'strong' and 'confident', fewer 'likes' were needed to dissipate their perceptions of oversharing anxieties. In turn, if they felt 'low' and 'weak', more 'likes' helped boost their self-esteem in the form of feedback. Interestingly, self-esteem was viewed as a mental state, which corresponded with a perceived physical state of strength and fitness. For example, low self-esteem was often expressed by feeling 'weak', and vice versa. Meanwhile, high self-esteem meant that they felt physically fit and strong. This highlights the relation of the mind–body continuum in regard to how users perceived their health; mental strength corresponded to feeling physically capable. The cartesian mind–body dualism is illustrated here, whereby the mind is perceived to be in control of the body and physical performance (Moore and Robinson, 2016). Furthermore, mental fragility contributed to feelings of doubt, whereby physical exercise goals were often felt unachievable, as demonstrated in Lara's case. She felt physically unfit and demotivated and posted about overcoming these barriers and managing to go for a run. She documented this by sharing a running selfie on Facebook, but she felt extremely anxious about sharing it as she felt it was unattractive:

> I didn't expect the amount of likes for my horrid running selfie, or such kind words, on Facebook. I nearly didn't post it there, but I'm glad I did now as it gave me a little boost and made me feel less shy or unable to post things in the future. I'm really conscious of overdoing it on FB 'cos I get annoyed with other people that do. (Lara, diary entry, 28, F)

In her final interview, on further examination of why she posted this when doing so made her feel so self-conscious, Lara explained that her reasoning was to break down expectations of 'perfect' fitness selfies that dominate social media. Lara wanted to reject and not conform to the dominant discourses and normalisations of representations of the body as a site of excellence (Gill and Scharff, 2011). She felt this image was more 'authentic' than the carefully sculpted, 'perfect' and sexualised images usually dominating Instagram (Elias and Gill, 2016), as she was slightly red in the face (because of the run) and squinting in the sunlight. In the caption, she also refers to the struggle to go out and run because she had a late night, drinking wine with friends, alluding to a hangover and highlighting the reality and ongoing balance of managing work, social life and exercise.

Most of the posts by users were carefully constructed in the conformist and objectified way; slim, fit bodies, styled food or beautiful locations become the key signifiers for representing healthy digital selves and healthy lifestyles. This carefully edited and stylised curation was a time-consuming and labour-intensive process, ironically as an attempt to appear 'in the moment'. However, these images become worth the time spent curating when enough 'likes' or positive feedback is received from the community in question.

> Today I posted a picture on Instagram of me at the gym after my boxing session. My motivation being to share progress of my 12-week challenge

> and how my muscle definition was coming along. Looking at the photo I feel proud of my progress so far and a big part of my motivation of sharing is to get feedback from people and I guess re-affirm to myself that I'm doing well. (...) One follower who commented 'foxy' is a personal trainer who has amazing arms so that made me feel good about myself (...) I've had a decent amount of likes of the image so far and all the time I spent editing and getting my gym friends to take a million pics for me to choose from was worth it! (Sophie, diary entry, 31, F)

> 'I'd be surprised, if I didn't get any responses.' (Roy, first interview, 26, M)

The users felt gratified by the positive feedback they gained from the community, which fed into their sense of 'health self' and identity. 'Enough' responses from the community can dissipate the sharer's anxiety. If enough 'likes' or positive responses are achieved, however subjectively that is interpreted, the potential for the voyeuristic gaze of the online community further encourages self-trackers sharing.

A 'like' for a 'like'!

As well as sharing their own data and health-related content, users also acknowledged that seeing other social media users sharing similar data and representations of being 'healthy' (such as gym or fitness photos) was also extremely motivating for them in their own practices:

> (On reflection) The other day I saw one of my Facebook friends had posted a run via run keeper [running app] so I wonder whether subconsciously this made me think to go for a run, so I could upload it too. (Sophie, diary entry, 31, F)

Seeing her friend posting about going for a run, when Sophie was not currently running as part of her own exercise routine, encouraged her to do the same. This was a common motivator for users to adopt different or new personal fitness routines. The users' surveying of others' posts on social media encourages them to take up not only comparable healthy behaviours but also ones that they can similarly capture and then share on social media to compete against others. Being accountable to the community, then, is a key motivator for the users to share their own health and fitness on social media and to publicly declare their activity through posts, which must then be maintained – a demonstration of 'sous-veillance' (Mann, 2013: 1), the 'many' (social media community) watching the few (users who post). This similarly reflects Foucault's (2008) identification of surveillance as a system of continual registration and inspection.

'Likes' become a form of emotional currency that contributes to a personal esteem for social media and self-tracking users. Acquisition of 'likes' provides the sharer with a sense of positive self-representation and reputation management. For example, Lara recommends somewhere 'healthy' for other local residents in Chamonix to eat, which builds her sense of self and identity as a fit, healthy and ethically engaged individual who supports local businesses. Adams and Raisborough (2008: 1166) identify how such practices work on the premise of a 'dynamic intersection of reflexivity, ethics, consumption and identity (...) of reflexive, concerned and known consumers'. Sharing these types of content attempts to encourage others towards similar 'healthy' practices and ethically driven, 'healthy' consumption practices. 'Likes' are expected to be received from regular sharers. As Forlano (2013: 6) explains: 'non-human artefacts are understood to be users in socio-technical systems in which they carry out specific "programs of action" in collaboration with humans.' These social media socio-technological affordances of 'likes' entwined user behaviours within these systems and technologies of the self, whereby gratification often relied on algorithmic sorting, working in the users' favour to gain 'likes':

> 'I managed to hit my target of 9 minutes, really chuffed to be able to post that. If I'm honest I think that post didn't get as many "likes" as I wanted on Facebook. I was like, "I didn't understand", I was like "maybe Facebook isn't working", 3 people liked it. When I was doing my marathon training, I was getting loads more likes (...) sometimes you're like, "I've just ran, like it."' (Sophie, final interview, 31, F)

If these representations of 'health' and reaching training goals were not positively received by the social media community in the form of 'likes', technology was blamed for not algorithmically prioritising a post and deep frustrations were felt in relation to the community for not recognising one's achievement. These annoyances also served as a reminder of the affordances and algorithmic influence of social media platforms (Thumin, 2012). Thus, the platform and its socio-technical elements were not serving its users in the way that the users served the platform and voluntarily shared data. Therefore, when the users recognised that these power relations were not reciprocal, they attempted tactical self-tracking and tactical sharing.

> I posted on this day because I haven't done so in a while and it's Valentine's day. I know a lot of people will be using Instagram today. (Fet, diary entry, 30, M)

Posting on Valentine's Day was a tactical move due to his assumption that many people would be sharing or 'showing off' photographs of their gifts on Instagram or indeed that the voyeurs would be privately surveying his content on this day. Fet's hope was that more people will be using the platform to post or scan content, even if this was likely centred around Valentine's Day, and therefore unrelated to 'health', so he still posted his cycling commute with the goal of gaining visibility. Although he did not have any data evidence, he perceived that there would be an increase in the number of users, who in turn would see and hopefully 'like' his content. Fet continuously felt assured that sharing data from his cycling commute was self-tracking for his own self-surveillance. At the end of the research period, on completing his diary reflections, Fet's perspectives shifted. In his final interview, he examined this progress and identified that gaining 'likes' impacted him a great deal:

> 'A lot of people are addicted to sharing, just like I used to post loads of things on Facebook (…) the more likes I got, the more sense of validation from other people (…) I guess with my cycling, I had probably posted for myself, but as I said I was going through this journey and I actually found myself liking the likes, (…) it certainly made me feel better that people knew that I was up at 6 in the morning doing the travel and managed to do the bike ride, people would sort of validate it, "oh he did 5 or so km in this time, that's pretty good."' (Fet, final interview, 30, M)

Fet identified gratification in two ways: firstly, feeling good for receiving 'likes' and, secondly, using 'likes' to provide motivation. As he expressed, he 'liked the likes'. They did indeed provide him with personal motivation to keep up his cycling commute, as well as motivation to track and share it. This difference between 'liking likes' and needing 'likes' to motivate cycling was examined in Lara's diary entry as well:

> I guess it depends on what mood you're in or what other interaction you have that day. I haven't posted anything in a few days, I'm still getting a few notifications from the posts though, likes and comments. It is a little boost, but I find it more curious too- are these genuine remarks or people trying to boost their own profile? I've been using social media but haven't really been actively taking part, apart from a few likes which isn't real interaction in my book. I'm craving seeing people more. (Lara, diary entry, 28, F)

Lara felt she did not need to post anything new as the 'likes' she was receiving from an earlier post were 'keeping her going'. Issues of trust and authenticity also came up when individuals were examining the role of 'likes' in their tracking and sharing practices: users often questioned if likes were genuine or not. The impossibility in determining the authenticity behind a 'like' (Marwick and boyd, 2010) became a core reasoning behind users considering them empty and void of emotional and social value. Further to this, written support on posts, private messages and telephone and face-to-face conversations were unsurprisingly deemed more authentic, genuine and valuable. The tangibility of particularly face-to-face contact with one's social circle or community was a key driver in users detoxing from their digital world, either by 'cutting down' or quitting and deleting social media permanently. Lou similarly felt that 'likes' only had so much traction; after some time and when other stresses in life such as work became dominating, 'likes' did not seem to hold as much value as when someone had time to track, share and survey:

> It's nice to touch base with them, with something more tangible than just a like. (Fet, diary entry, 30, M)

> 'Up to a point with training you need a bit of encouragement, and you need a bit of almost normal people who aren't running a marathon telling you that what you're doing is impressive and then you're like "ah yeah, it is, thanks." After a while you're just like "actually, I've got to finish this sodding marathon."' (Lou, final interview, 29, F)

For users training towards specific goals, feedback from the community in the form of 'likes' held only limited value and motivation. Though users associated their online community with a sense of sociality and support, they felt that something was missing, notably a genuine validation of their achievements by peers who shared other interests, who may have eased the burden of a surveillant gaze. In sum, the currency of 'likes' offers only a one-dimensional transaction and source of emotional nourishment for self-trackers over extended periods of time.

Conclusions

The datafication and quantification of health have led to an economic climate of personal health data becoming a capitalist commodity. The personalisation that arises from datafication and digital phenotyping is a form of surveillance by tech, state and online social media communities. Data has become a regular currency for citizens, users and patients to pay for their communication services and use of these platforms. Arguably, this has become further normalised since COVID-19 contact tracing applications and other surveillance methods for monitoring and managing public health; this is further examined in Chapter 7, 'Future Directions for the Digital Health Self'. Risk profiling via digital phenotyping, or even via less opaque forms of surveillance, means tech giants and even insurance companies can monitor us through our wearable tech or our social media behaviours. Surveillance of health practices can be captured into digitally quantifiable (Lupton 2012) as well as qualitative formats. What is perhaps most alarming, at least in the context of the analyses in this book, is that datafication of health is rooted in problematic claims of revolutionising healthcare, individually and for public and population health. Dataism (van Dijck, 2014), as a concept to conceive these phenomena in a critical light, illustrates the widespread belief that personal data is entrusted to corporate platforms for the public and personal good. This problematic notion of trust from citizens, consumers and patients increasingly interlocks government, tech and wellness industries and private and public healthcare sectors into an ecosystem of networked actors, each with their own commercial incentive and vested interest to capture, mine and monetise our personal data for health purposes. Additionally, self-trackers embody this logic in their everyday lives, which promotes the idea that acquiring more data is better for health analysis regardless of health outcomes, whereby the choice architecture and 'nudging' design of health apps further cement these mechanised performances of human capacity through the designed incentives of behavioural economics that are embedded in these platforms. This logic promotes a practice for the digital healthy self, even subconsciously; of a proactive mind, separate from a bodily response. Here, the body responds to the device – an arguable automation – in an assemblage whereby the symbiotic agency prioritises bodily regulation and automation, when, at times, this might be to the detriment of personal, physical or mental health.

3

Surveillance Cultures of the Digital Health Self

This chapter explores the role of surveillance when health is managed by and performed with the use of self-tracking and social media technologies in everyday life. By sharing health-related content on social media, users become representative of a community of like-minded 'health'-orientated individuals, which they – even when nothing is being personally achieved – feel a part of. This is illustrated through the analysis of the empirical data, interviews, reflexive diaries and online content. This chapter explores how these practices positively and optimistically contribute to users' sense of self and identity as informed, productive and improving 'healthy' beings, reflecting surveillance capitalism's techno-utopian ideologies in promoting the use of these platforms for sociality and as a tool for self and peer surveillance (Tufecki, 2008; boyd and Hargittai, 2010; Trottier, 2012; Lupton, 2014; Zuboff, 2019). Whilst this book recognises surveillance capitalism as the 'new economic order that claims human experience as free raw material for hidden commercial practices of extraction, prediction, and sales' (Zuboff, 2015: np), this chapter predominantly focuses upon the impact of this logic on users (that is, consumers). These self-tracking and social media platforms tend to obfuscate their economic practices, techno-commercial infrastructures and strategies (Moore and Robinson, 2016; Moore, 2017; Srincek, 2017; van Dijck et al, 2018; Lupton, 2019; Zuboff, 2019), whilst prompting and promoting users to engage and share their lifestyles, frequently presented as self-empowerment, personal optimisation and life improvement. Through the logic of surveillance capitalism, the economic infrastructures and extraction of value from data become opaque, and this lack of transparency mitigates further engagement via neoliberal self-responsibilising and betterment strategies. The integral role of community surveillance is examined in how users' self-survey with social media and self-tracking tools. This is often in consideration to how their social media community online may perceive them (imagined surveillance), the important role of feedback (or lack of), which pervasively reinforces these individuals' sense of health self and continual engagement with these platforms of tools of surveillance.

This chapter also examines shifts in sharing practices under considerations of self and community surveillance; for example, when individuals experience stress or trauma in their personal lives, this often leads to concealment of 'unhealthy' behaviours to avoid the negative judgement of others online. This also relieves users from being the object of the communities' gaze and judging their own lives through comparing lifestyles represented and surveilled on social media. This chapter highlights how the accumulative and collaborative information produced through these platforms changes users' behaviours and understandings of their bodies and health, which are reinforced by the (lack of) feedback received from their social media communities (Kent, 2018). Surveillance and privacy issues are analysed within the context of digital performativity and management of the 'digital health self'.

Digital health self under surveillance

Since the seventeenth century, technologies of measurement have been tools that have provided legitimacy and with it an authority in managing people and populations (Nafus and Sherman, 2014). The information technology revolution of the twentieth century made it possible to govern individuals and cities through various surveillance methods (Townsend, 2013). These practices of measuring populations are 'entangled with the practices of measuring and disciplining bodies' (Nafus and Sherman, 2014 4). The production of authority and the disciplining of populations and various bodies are exercised through, for example, the national census, which identifies the population size and demographics, discerning 'people who count from those who do not' (Scott, 1998). Poovey (1998: np) outlines how it was the 'fledgling business class who first effectively mobilised the gravitas of scientific rationality to legitimise commerce by creating distance between the measured and the measurer'. This distancing between the measured and the measurer, enabled through 'merchants' early accounting techniques, turned into vast and elaborate tools of state control' (Nafus and Sherman, 2014: 2) and first evoked big data ideologies of cataloguing, systematisation, quantification and making useful knowledge about the world.

The digital health self is under surveillance in everyday life – surveillance of oneself (self-surveillance) surveillance of and by others (online and offline) to benchmark healthy or unhealthy practices and digital surveillance enabled by social media and self-tracking devices to monitor the body, as well as practices of surveillance capitalism and data mining of personal data across digital platforms. The reasons and rationale for these practices vary hugely, which this chapter speaks to throughout; however, for analytical focus this first section explores perceived positive motivations for surveillant practices of the health self. According to Whitson and Haggerty (2008: 574), online self-presentation occurs where 'citizens are encouraged, enticed and occasionally compelled into bringing components of their fractured and dispersed data double into regular patterns of contact, scrutiny and management'. Surveillance, therefore, becomes a 'system of constant registration and constant inspection' (Goodyear et al, 2017: 3).

Inspection through health monitoring using apps, by the users as well as community surveillance online, is a cyclical process of self-analysis, performativity and reflection. Lyon (2003: 20) understands surveillance as a system that 'obtains personal and group data in order to classify people and populations according to varying criteria, to determine who should be targeted for special treatment, suspicion, eligibility, inclusion, access, and so on'. This book identifies the role of surveillance for self-trackers as a personal practice that is technologically enabled, state-driven and fiercely monetised by digital and platform capitalism.

Surveillance, in this book, is a concept that is certainly not innocent or neutral. It is a tool that is at times voluntarily embodied (self-surveillance), at times used as a performance for the gaze of others (peer/community surveillance). Yet in both cases it is used to exercise power. Self-surveillance through devices and apps is presented as offering agency (Mann, 2005), which could be perceived as a rejection of state or top-down supervision. However, their voluntary use plays directly into the hands of their makers, who capitalise and profit from their use. Why then do users feel the desire to share these fragments of their data selves and what do they gain from such sharing of personal information and lifestyles? It is doubtful whether users consider the impact of 'surveillance capitalism' and its entailment of privacy threats and 'opaque forms of datafied power and domination' (Kristensen and Ruckenstein, 2018: 3). As Davies (2016: 196) argues, 'networks have a tendency towards what are called "power laws", whereby those with influence are able to harness that power to win even greater influence.' The power of influence here, I align with the platform developers in their prioritisation and capitalisation of surveillance, as well as users' awareness of the important role of the surveillance of others regarding what they post, on which platform and why. Users' perceptions and management of their own visibility online and the visibility of others are tied to shifting understandings of what is considered public and private personal data and information. Online communities and social media 'organise relations between peers. Not only are interpersonal social ties mediated on an organisational platform, but interpersonal activity also becomes asynchronous. Peer relations become more surveillant in nature' (Trottier, 2012: 320). It then becomes important to consider how the surveillance of others influences users self-presentation, especially with the continually evolving and shifting socio-technological affordances and understandings of both self-tracking technologies and social media.

The ambiguous health goal of self-betterment

Self-trackers do not always outline a specific goal but are curious about the information implied by the acquired numbers and data (Wolf, 2010). Therefore, as Langwieser and Kirig (2010: 105) argue: 'the rules of our knowledge-based meritocracy invite to this self-optimisation: Who wants to be healthy, happy and successful, needs to become a self-designer.' 'Self-designing' to achieve health goals is illustrative of the healthism discourses, tied to ideals of self-betterment and 'optimisation' promoted by the tech, fitness and wellness industries. Situating this narrative within the socio-economic and political underpinnings of neoliberalism, we see a wide ideological shift within society now, from viewing the individual as a 'passive' patient and consumer of healthcare to viewing them as 'active' consumer of healthcare (Tritter, 2009).

> 'I've always just wanted to be the best version I can be so I'm always looking at what I can do, it's always been kind of drummed in, I don't know where it's come from but there's always, what can I do better, or what could I have done differently.' (Lara, final interview, 28, F)

> 'If you go to a gym everybody is there for self-improvement so that's a better place to train.' (Roy, final interview, 26, M)

Motivation towards self-improvement through surveillance of one's own health and fitness behaviours is often the initial reason for starting to use a self-tracker. Yet users often recognised that they did not know why they felt this way. Preventing ill health, disease or death was surprisingly infrequently identified or discussed as a reason for managing and improving personal health. The discourses that surround health self-care and individualised and privatised health practices, advocated by the state and lifestyle health and wellness apps, assume that people have the power to choose healthy or unhealthy lifestyles. Therefore, integration of these tools translates 'relationships between people, ideas, and things into algorithms in order to engineer and steer performance' (van Dijck, 2013b: 202). Steering self-improvement via surveillance enabled by health apps provides a sense of personal control for individuals taking charge of and authority over proactive health changes – not always, however, to reach specific goals:

> I believe that my current health is good; I am in good shape so therefore calorie counting and losing weight is not my priority. I am more focused on speed and being in a better shape. (Fet, diary entry, 30, M)

Often, self-betterment health goals were highly ambiguous and non-definitive about what self-improvement meant for these users. Rather, they simply articulated that the goal was to optimise the body, based on the belief that the more we understand ourselves through tech interventions to increase 'health status', the more we can improve ourselves (Noji et al, 2021: 261). Though human beings have done this for centuries with analogue methods and diarising (Walker-Rettberg, 2018) and through technologies of quantification and surveillance such as self-tracking applications, these become 'technologies of the self' (Foucault, 1988). This discourse translates ideas of identification of the self into the prevention or cure of health issues, which can provide an 'economy of hope' (Novas, 2006: 289). These political and promissory economies of hope (Novas, 2006; Rose, 2007) present the logics of optimisation and improvement as an attainable goal and form of control through personal diagnosis, self-tracking and the 'hopeful' prevention of pathologies. Arguably, this could be understood as contributing to the proliferation of the 'worried well', whereby the continual monitoring and capturing of data about the body through self-tracking devices and associated practices provoke unneeded anxiety in those who are 'healthy' (Husain and Spence, 2015: 2). In this regard, the 'worried well' self-triggers health anxieties through an over-examination of the body and health via these technologies. Thus, what manifests itself is a drive to continually 'optimise' and 'improve' health to feel productive, proactive and therefore 'healthy', thus enacting care of the self and responsible citizenship practices (Rose, 1999):

> 'I like improvement and seeing things getting better, not necessarily getting to the best in that thing but to get to see the progression in myself. Like, that's where I started and either that's what I can do or that's what I couldn't do and then to work for it, put in hard work and the rewards of it are purely in my own mind and body. It's not for any other kind of greater gain, not to look better or for anyone's opinions of me to be any different. It's just that I feel really good that I've started somewhere. I worked hard, I looked into stuff and I improved. That's the main gain for me.' (Tim, final interview, 35, M)

Bio-political dimensions of the digital health self

Bio-politics, as briefly introduced in Chapter 1, refers to techniques of governance over a population as a political problem; that is, it is at once scientific and biological as well as about the politics of power (Foucault, 1979b: 245). As Foucault expands (1979b: 252–253) expands:

> To say that power took possession of life in the nineteenth century (...) is to say that it has, thanks to the play of technologies of discipline on

> the one hand and technologies of regulation on the other, succeeded in covering the whole surface that lies between the organic and the biological, between body and population. We are, then, in a power that has taken control of both the body and life or that has, if you like, taken control of life in general – with the body as one pole and the population as the other.

In a neoliberal society, individuals are positioned as consumers of health expected to take personal responsibility and education to maintain individual self-care. Non-commodified public spheres such as healthcare are being replaced by commercial systems through encouraging the adoption of self-tracking devices, which serve to enable self-regulatory monitoring behaviours. Self-identifying is therefore achieved through self-transformation, as well as life-strategising technologies of the self to compete within a community, which is further encouraged through self-tracking applications and practices (Urry and Elliot, 2010).

> 'I still want to keep pushing myself as best I can with regards to the fitness thing. I've still got goals I want to achieve before it's physically impossible for me to achieve them. It's always going to be a part of my life I think.' (Matt, final interview, 41, M)

These active practices of self-care situated these individuals as 'active' consumers and participators of 'health', with choice being the key mechanism used to promote individuals as consumers within health care systems (Tritter, 2009).

> [D]iscourses of digitised health promotion position digital technologies as providing the obvious solutions to social and economic problems. [Holding] out the promise of control (…) over the unruly population who are viewed as making ever-greater demands on the health system and the budget of governments. (Lupton, 2013c: 14–15)

Lupton (2013c) identifies one of the key issues around self-tracking and quantification: its practice in relation to bio-politics, state and corporate surveillance and monetisation of personal data. This book understands 'biometrics as a technology of biopower whereby the body and life itself are the subject of modalities of control, regimes of truth, and techniques of sorting and categorisation' (Ajana, 2013: 5). It must, therefore, be recognised that whatever is being captured by these devices is biased towards whatever a particular population wants to capture, or the business model of the specific tech company profiting from surveillance capitalism (Zuboff, 2019). As Nafus and Sherman (2014: 1) argue: 'The QS [quantified self] movement attracts both the most hungrily panoptic of data aggregation business, and people who have developed their own notions of analytics that are separate from and in relation to dominant practices of firms and institutionalised scientific production.' Rose (2009: 11) similarly acknowledges that medicine is reshaped by 'requirements of public or private insurance, their criteria for reimbursement (…) treatment of health and illness as merely another field for calculations of corporate profitability'. The role of national capital and state priorities, therefore, directs and informs public health:

> Bio-politics does not intervene in a therapeutic way, nor does it seek to individualise or modify a person (this would entail the production of subjectivity itself). Instead, it functions at the level of generality with the aim to identify risk groups, risk factors, and risk levels, and therefore anticipate, prevent, contain and manage potential risk. (Foucault, 2003: 235–236)

Foucault (2003) here identifies how bio-politics does not take into consideration individual subjectivities but operates at a wider level, demonstrating a passage from disciplinary to control societies (Lazzarato, 2006: 171). This is what makes 'bio-power more effective and less obtrusive' (Rose, 1999: 236). As Ajana (2005: 3) astutely observes: 'without subjectivity, the possibility of resistance fades into the immanent arrangements and administrative operations of bio-politics.' If bio-politics does not acknowledge subjectivity but operates through state-wide subtle rationalities, how can an individual or the public resist or reject dominant systems? This becomes 'part and parcel of responsibilisation through which individuals are made in charge of their behaviour, competence, improvement, security, and well-being' (Ajana, 2005: 3). Such a proliferation of systemic dominance over the public becomes embodied, and bio-politics therefore becomes effective: 'the maintenance of the healthy body [has become] central to self-management of many individuals and families, employing practices ranging from dietetics and exercise, through to the consumption of proprietary medicines and health supplements, to self-diagnosis and treatment' (Rose, 1999: 10). In neoliberal societies, self-surveillance as a means of self-managing health is a common feature of proactive citizenship responsibilities. Being on a self-betterment 'journey' to achieve better health and individual skill development was a dominant discourse in all the participants' diary entries and final interviews, in which digital platforms enabled the space to look back and forward. Reaching 'peaks' of expertise in one practice motivated individuals to vary their exercises, and thus enabled further development and self-bettering, with 'choice' and 'opportunity' referred to as tools for motivating new exercise regimes or health-related lifestyle changes.

> 'I'll always find something else. I'll get something in my head that I want to do, I'll do that and then I'll move on to the next thing. I'm always striving to go on to the next step. Running I'll set a time, I'll get that PB and I'll want to go faster, it's the same with everything I do (...) it's just a constant learning cycle with it, you're never not learning I suppose.' (Matt, final interview, 41, M)

Learning, optimising and improving became a continual cycle of enactment and desire (Viseu and Suchman, 2010), regardless of where it would take the participants and irrespective of specific end goals. They subsequently considered it to be a responsible process. In sum, within the discourse of self-surveillance and self-managing health behaviours exists a core pressure to be 'active' and to perform 'healthy' behaviours, to 'optimise' health. This leads to a sense of personal success, pride and elation.

Pride in self-surveillance and self-tracking

Increased health awareness is part of the shift within healthcare from a public, state and medical responsibility frame to a private responsibility frame (Lawrence, 2004), whereby individuals are encouraged to manage their own health through increased individual self-knowledge (Lupton, 2012a). This shift in health responsibility ensures that individuals and patients now continually look towards (new) media, platforms and digital health technologies to obtain (mis)information about health (King and Watson, 2005), symptomatic analysis, nutritional and lifestyle advice, illness prevention and even healthcare policy (Seale, 2003). This reinforces the dominant perspective of self-trackers, that their sense of satisfaction and pride in self-surveillance and tracking is further rationalised as a means of effectively self-managing their own healthcare (Green and Hubbard, 2012):

> I felt like my good result gave me more energy, as I felt over the moon. I'd accomplished something personally. I was certainly full of energy today at work. (Fet, diary entry, 30, M)

Similarly, individualised control is often seen as a positive manifestation of self-management, related to the perceived 'ease' of using the application. Here is a visible reflection of QS movement discourses: 'if you cannot measure it, you cannot improve it' (Kelly, 2011: np). This techno-celebratory discourse asserts that commitment to and practices of self-surveillance and monitoring of personal bodily functions will improve physical health. This research extends this perspective, in that pride in self-tracking and gaining a good 'time' or 'result' additionally contributes to positive mental health and feelings of personal 'energy' that genuinely motivate user and very interestingly manifests as a physical energy:

> Well over my daily step goal today, so relatively happy. (Matt, diary entry, 41, M)

> I feel motivated to try and beat the time and average speed of my previous journey, a competition with myself. (Fet, diary entry, 30, M)

Users' perceptions of their own happiness became linked with reaching or exceeding self-tracking goals, understood as a competition with oneself and considered as a positive motivation for improving fitness. Furthermore, self-tracking proved to be helpful and supportive for being accountable to oneself. The motivation to self-track was not always to reach any set goal but rather just to know that one was continually improving in whatever way that was subjectively interpreted. This could be interpreted in Kevin Kelly's (co-founder of the QS movement) techno-utopian terms, which argue that 'quantifying yourself is an act of self-assertion. All this attention is not a narcissist adoration of the self, but a self-definition in an age of great uncertainty about who we are' (2011: np). For a time, beating personal goals through self-tracking practices made the users feel productive or active and contributed to their sense of identity as improving 'healthy' beings. Individualised 'consumption (practices) have become the primary site for self-identification (…) in which taste and appearance are seen to be deployed as the basis of evaluative judgments of a person's moral worth and their social position' (Adams and Raisborough, 2008: 1173). A sense of moral worth is often achieved through attaining personal health goals:

> I felt really good and wanted to keep up the good routine of running regularly, doing more yoga and eating well. My mood was really good, I felt real sense of myself, like my confidence from the commitment I was making to myself was reassuring me somehow. (Lara, diary entry, 28, F)

This confidence ascribed to meeting goals, Adams and Raisborough (2008) argue, is achieved through two sociological considerations: that the self is now being predisposed to relentlessly engage in a (self-) reflexive practice (Giddens, 1991) and that consumption practices have now emerged as the 'privileged site' for such identity work (Adams and Raisborough, 2008: 1166). This perspective was reflected in multiple user accounts:

> I do find the more I make time for myself, the stronger I feel in myself to cope with other things. I find it really head clearing and affirmative in my own decision making. (Lara, diary entry, 28, F)

> 'I was thinking, this is something I have to stick with now, when I am stressed, don't just go to the pub and moan about it with a bottle of wine. Say no and put on your running shoes and run home. You're never going to regret that.' (Lou, final interview, 29, F)

Control and self-discipline over the body, routines, health and fitness-related practices make the user feel 'stronger' in themselves as well as empowered (Banner, 2012). These feelings become embodied and woven into the fabric of the prideful digital health self. This commitment to self-governance was often interpreted by the participants as an everyday habit, frequently identified as a motivation to maintain, improve and optimise 'health' for those that had been integrating related practices into their routine for many years.

Traversing agential boundaries: competition with oneself and one's device

Pride in personal surveillance and health tracking achieved by reaching personal goals, according to the research findings, additionally binds self-trackers to the self-monitoring task for further personal development. Where can one go once personal goals are achieved? Well, the next self-improvement strategy demonstrated was competition with oneself. Self-trackers hitting personal targets turn towards further self-improvement, highlighting bio-political discourses of responsibilisation (Foucault, 1979b; Rose, 2007; Ajana, 2013), the self-regulation in which individuals are encouraged and incited to become new active consumers of continuous healthcare, taking personal responsibility and educating themselves as a means of maintaining personal improvement:

> I felt a sense of competitiveness with myself as there are certain yoga poses I want to achieve, and I can feel from practicing more regularly they're more within reach now. (Lara, diary entry, 28, F).

> Personally, I want to keep a track of everything I'm doing. Running is a big part of what I do so it's become almost habitual. (Lou, diary entry, 29, F).

Self-trackers measure self-improvement through the systems of measurement on digital health apps. However, they also exist but in a less visible form in the measurement of personal development through surveillance governance: the use of these technologies to perceive their digital health self-improvement and development. The concern is not always to 'share' this data, practice or development, but rather pride is felt in the perceived management of the self, achieved through performed and embodied self-governance to 'achieve' and generate data, regardless of results. The 'sense' of feeling one is continually improving becomes the individual system of measurement and regulation of the body. For example, Tim pushed himself to do yoga practice when he was very unwell:

> You would probably say this was typical of me… Practically dying with flu and a chest infection but still hiking off through snow covered woods, to a lake, to do yoga… Sense of self ticked :). (Tim, diary entry, 34, M)

Tim expanded on this perspective in his final interview, when he asserted that even though he was extremely unwell he had to do his yoga practice, quite simply because he 'always did it'. Tim's internal system of measurement of maintaining continual improvement was daily yoga practice, regulated and maintained regardless of ill health and infection. In discussions around the question of whether users would not exercise if they were unwell or too tired, most acknowledged that they would still continue with their usual regimes. Interestingly, this is perceived as 'automatic' due to habit and commitment to training programmes as an authority of control:

> 'That doesn't happen, literally never ever. I'll be like screw you we're going training anyway (…) It's just habit, like my brain will go I'm tired, It's a force of habit. It doesn't cost any energy to get up and train anyway. It's what you do. It's like going to work.' (Roy, final interview, 26, M)

> Personally, I want to keep a track of everything I'm doing. Running is a big part of what I do so it's become almost habitual. (Lou, diary entry, 29, F)

> 'Don't feel like I decided to work out today. That's what the programme says, so I do it. It's quite essential to put the programme in front and stick to it for a certain period of time, then have the set moment where you evaluate and go: did this work; yes or no (…) For that reason, you have to stick to a programme consistently for a while before you see results. Two weeks abs don't exist. You'll barely see any noticeable progress in two weeks.' (Roy, final interview, 26, M)

Not just part of user's daily routine, the tracking and following training programmes also become a tangible authority figure for self-trackers. It is important to acknowledge here how 'matter and meaning are mutually articulated' (Barad, 2007: 152) through this onto-epistemological process of being with and living through our devices. As Karen Barad continues, 'agency is not an attribute but the ongoing reconfiguring's of the world' (2003: 813); thus, this navigation between self-tracker and device is negotiated by a continual balance being addressed in agential terms. On the one hand, the self-tracker motivated by pride in self-surveillance enacts health improvement practices (exercising or eating well), and on the other, the health app itself is seen a tool of agency and power over the users' behaviour monitoring and surveilling them. Training programmes can be conceptualised as a disciplinary regime, a habitual process and productive activity of the digital health self in the digital society of today. Self-trackers do not always feel they 'decide' to work out; they do it because their 'programme says so'. Fitness regimes and programmes are in command; these technologies and techniques of the self (Foucault, 1988) dictate behaviours that push and guide individuals' health practices. Further discussions in the final interviews resonated with this idea, that this sense of technologically shaped self-governance directed users' behaviours. The individual and the body operate in a mechanical fashion. One could consider this a voluntary willingness to follow set goals through an exercise, diet or general lifestyle regime with rules and boundaries. As many users concede, this practice reinforces one's sense of self through self-discipline and self-regulation. Unpacking this through a proposal of 'response-ability' – the ability to respond – Barad argues that our range of responses to a device are conditioned by and through practices of engagement (in Kleinman, 2018). If I apply this theorisation of responding to a nudge from our self-tracking app to follow a training programme, for example, what the device is doing is presenting the human user with an obligation to follow it. In other words, 'responsibility is an iterative (re)opening up to an enabling of responsiveness' (Barad in Kleinman, 2018: 81). To respond to a self-tracker in this way can conceivably be seen as a conditioning exemplified by the users in the research findings. To speak in techno-utopian terms, this could provide the users with a sense of a 'health' identity and personal meaning, which actively contributes to individual narratives (Giddens, 1991) of proactive health management. The individual responds with subjectivity arguably removed from the process of meaning-making, as they engage in automated, tech-directed behaviours.

On the other hand, this could be considered an extension of the neoliberal 'government of the soul' (Rose, 1999: 11), which is in line with self-improvement discourses that advocate self-betterment as the dominant priority during 'rest' periods (for example, holidays) or when unwell. In this case, exercise may in fact not be 'good' for the user. In contrast, training routines and exercising are also perceived as a desired structure and self-disciplinary practice, viewed as a way to escape demands related to work and social life, but a disciplinary and tiresome routine not always mentally wanted or physically needed. This viewpoint arguably emerges in response to broader socio-cultural and political neoliberal discourses related to the betterment, improvement and optimisation of the self through technology (Moore and Robinson, 2016; Moore, 2017). The priority here, then, is the focus on being productive and improving oneself. For self-trackers this often became the individual identity, identifier and embodiment of feeling like an ethical citizen, consumer or individual, regardless of any actual developments or whether this was in fact to the detriment of their physical or mental health. Arguably, in this way, these training regimes or self-betterment goals were imposed and adhered to as a form of dealing with individual uncertainties about their own lives (Giddens, 1991), futures and health. Control, therefore, for these users was enabled by aspirations towards and ideals of how best to manage and improve health management and self-betterment. To step outside of and resist these frames of self-governance would be to resist panoptic surveillance (Foucault 1979), presented through the consumer devices and broader governing discourses of being a morally 'good' proactive individual and citizen (this is further examined in Chapter 4). This chimes with Foucault's (1979, 1997b: 67) concept of 'governmentality': the regulatory activity that shapes the self as well as public beliefs and behaviours surrounding health maintenance and self-management. The parameters and goals set by the individuals within these technologies illustrate Moore and Robinson's (2016: 2776) conceptualisation of neoliberalism as 'an affective regime exposing a risk of assumed subordination of bodies to technologies'. This affective regime of the body to technology is a key regulation advocated and enabled through self-tracking devices as well as competitive and comparative representations on social media.

Self-representation and expected community surveillance

Public and private binary distinctions are often insufficient for describing online (health) communities. Interpersonal surveillance is considered a violation but also to be a pervasive condition of social media. This 'intervisibility' (Brighenti, 2010) ensures that interpersonal surveillance is mutual, whereby privacy violations are normalised through visibility of shared content of personal health. Users now understand, arguably, that there is a 'trade off' between managing privacy and achieving public exposure (Tufecki, 2008; boyd and Hargittai, 2010). Within these online platforms users 'put on their daily lives as staged performances where they deliberately use the differentiation between private and public discursive acts to shape their identity. Each construction of self entails a strategy aimed at performing a social act or achieving a particular social goal' (van Dijck, 2013b: 212), social media self-presentation then, we can see as a salient narrative of the technologically mediated life in the digital society of today. Furthermore, as Moore (2017: np) contends, 'capitalism, as the current global political economic model within which we live, is becoming a system of increasingly empty selves, subject to unending capitalist social reproduction, where data simply confirms the order, it has already prefabricated.' Keen (2015: np) takes a particularly dystopian perspective and considers the internet as structurally parochial: 'like a village (…) we're all clustering in these tighter and tighter ideological and cultural networks. There's no serendipity, no stumbling upon random people or random ideas. Everything is pre-ordained; you're served with what you know will suit you.' Similarly, Brabazon (2015: 62) argues that the parochial nature of social media informs the communicative practices and interpersonal relations online at a particular moment in time 'the dominant media of a time influences the type of empire constructed'. Although media has always provided a window into the private life of others (Meyrowitz, 1986), Trottier (2012: 321) considers social networks and lateral 'surveillance is more than data collection because it relies on mediated relations, profiling and asymmetrical relations of visibility. It is the dominant organisational logic of late modernity' (Trottier, 2012: 320). In this regard, if surveillance and organisational profiling are conditions of contemporary society in the digital age, interpersonal and lateral surveillance have increasingly become accepted as the norm.

As was explored in Chapter 2, with self-tracking practices, the relationship between health and data becomes intrinsically linked. This leads to a 'datafication of health' (Ruckenstein and Schull, 2017: 262) as data becomes the significant tangible evidence for users' self-betterment and achievements. For the participants in these research projects, health data regularly held more significance than personal self-gratification, for 'seeing' this produced data felt more 'factual' and 'credible' than the physical acts or exercise that produced it (Ruckenstein, 2014). Once self-tracking devices capture the data representation of the body, the feedback from the device causes the user to be continually aware of their own bodily moments, but once shared on social media, others' gaze may increase pressures upon the user to change or adapt their lifestyle for the viewing community. For example, Nigel has been regularly running at the weekend and sharing his data on Facebook:

> 'I had a situation where I went for a run at the weekend and then came back and didn't post anything and somebody asked me: "Didn't you go for a run this weekend?" So, that was interesting. I just forgot to post it.' (Nigel, first interview, 49, M)

Nigel expanded that this message came from an old acquaintance and Facebook 'Friend' via a private message on Facebook Messenger. He explained that he had not seen this acquaintance for many years; he had never publicly fed back or 'liked' any of his previous running posts. This other user and 'voyeur' was privately viewing Nigel's content but never publicly feeding back on it on the platform. Nigel reflected that he was now more inclined to not only ensure he kept running but also share his data with the now-known imagined community, who were privately viewing but not publicly feeding back. This supports boyd's (2014: 4) assertion that online participation becomes 'entirely normal, even expected'; if you regularly share health-related data, this then becomes expected by the wider social media community of followers. Nigel's example illustrates David Lyon's theory of 'liquid surveillance',

> [which situates] surveillance developments in the fluid and unsettling modernity of today. Surveillance softens, especially in the consumer realm. Old moorings are loosened as bits of personal data extracted for one purpose are more easily deployed in another. Surveillance spreads in hitherto unimaginable ways, responding to and reproducing liquidity. (2013: 2–3)

This fluid and unexpected surveillance by and of these users meant routines were then altered to enable time for certain exercise or health practices that could be tracked and shared online now that the data had become liquid, viewed by unknown surveilling audience. Similarly, in the reverse this consciousness of observations from others within the community can also encourage self-censoring or the concealment of practices, ensuring 'unhealthy' practices are not shared on social media (or at all):

> 'You can kind of see the frequency of people's posts. If they normally post food photos and they haven't for a while then it's probably because they're eating rubbish.' (Jennie, first interview, 40, F)

Posting is expected from regular sharers, and if not performed, this can be considered as indicative of 'unhealthy' behaviours or a lack of self-tracking and health improvement. This is also interpreted as a lack of commitment from the self-tracker, as not being in line with discourses of self-regulation and discipline to achieve improvement or health optimisation. This neoliberal 'government of the soul' (Rose, 1999: 11) ensures that the judgemental discourse attached to being inactive ('lazy') encourages individuals to undertake self-surveillance practices and to prioritise self-management over health by actively undertaking 'healthy' behaviours. The continual presence of the communities' gaze, combined with regulatory processes of monitoring personal (in)action, marks this type of surveillance as a deeply embedded and persistent influence (Webb and Quennerstedt, 2010). Not being 'there' and visible for your community was a feeling that all of the participants felt at some point during the research period. This guilt was attached not just to a lack of commitment to healthy goals but also to the decision not to post. Not posting could therefore be seen as indicative of censored unhealthy behaviours, as Jennie demonstrated, because the community expects you to post, to maintain social interaction and to keep them updated. Therefore, the networked audience becomes 'a collaborator in the identity and content presented by the speaker, and the imagined audience becomes visible when it influences the information (...) users choose to broadcast' (Marwick and boyd, 2010: 17). This collaborative dynamic develops into feelings of pressure to be visible to others:

> [I feel] guilty for not posting much and annoyed as I will be losing followers and traffic through my platforms. (Annie, diary entry, 28, F)

> Felt a bit like I had to share something on Instagram... even though the run wasn't all that picturesque – bit stressful to be honest thinking about needing to take a photo on the run. Gave up once I started getting tired and remembered this wasn't why I'm running! (Lou, diary entry, 29, F)

Users expected community surveillance as part and parcel of data-sharing cultures and often experienced this as a form of stress associated with their fitness or health practices: to maintain their set goals and to document and share this regularly with their social media community for the communities' benefit and not just their own. This 'imposed self-tracking' (Lupton, 2016b: 103) and 'participatory surveillance' (Albrechtslund and Lauritsen, 2008: 310) over time felt too invasive. Therefore, I identify the detrimental pressures that using these platforms places upon users. The 'precise articulation of property rights calibrates the control exercised over the flow of data. Intellectual property law and user agreements are key regulations that guarantee the controlled flow of BSD [Big Social Data] through a highly proprietary environment' (Cote, 2014: 138). The majority of self-tracking applications and data capture devices are access, not ownership, models (Swan, 2012a). As Cote (2014) acknowledges, users may generate 'social data' but as soon as it enters the human and non-human assemblage, whether this be online or offline, the proprietor is no longer solely the user who generated it, but still the pressure to generate it pervasively exists.

Competition and comparison in community surveillance

Surveillance of other users' social media accounts and sharing online affected the participants' own health practices (Ziebland and Wyke, 2012). This voyeurism was identified as a common community practice on social media and was employed as a competitive and comparative tool. For all the participants, achieving certain goals either individually or competitively within the community was considered 'good enough' to be shared because it demonstrated individual improvement. For sharers, this voyeurism was also identified as a community practice enabling competition and comparisons with other users. Using self-tracking and social media platforms can provide a dual function: users self-track, quantify and record their health practices, and they can also observe and compare themselves with others, which in turn motivate and inform their health choices. As demonstrated by Sophie:

> 'The app would tell me afterwards if you'd set a record, so you could share that on social media. There'd often be challenges as well, and you could see what your friends were doing with leader boards.' (Sophie, first interview, 31, F)

Social media sites, therefore, through their algorithmically organised sociality channels, ensure that personal meritocracy is disciplined through achievement ranking. As discussed earlier in the chapter, this is accomplished through the quantification of feedback or 'likes' on social media as well as through community leadership boards on self-tracking apps. I liken this competition to gaining recognition or positive feedback online within scoring systems of measurement, which encapsulate a 'feedback economy' and a metrification of status (Marwick and boyd, 2010). Furthermore, in Ajana's (2013: 21) terms, I can see this as the 're-mediation of measurement', whereby status becomes quantifiable through data statistics. For instance, Lara was running a 10 km run in Chamonix, which included a huge elevation of running up and down a mountain. Other friends of hers were doing the same route with varying distances of up to 80 km:

> 'I was noting other people that weekend that had done the marathon. It was really motivating to watch them. They were all posting their times, but I didn't post my time because, what I shared, it was honest but there were bits that were missing, I didn't want to admit how long it took me. I was proud of the fact that I'd done it, but I didn't want anyone else to judge how long it took me. About comparing, the 10 km was the lowest race you could do. The day before there had been an 80 km race, and it's not just 80 kms, it's fricking up and down the mountain as well. It was proper effort, but it felt like proper effort for me as well, but I felt like it wasn't the same.' (Lara, final interview, 28, F)

Apart from the judgement of posts, this competition between social media members can operate as a tool for comparable as well as unintended surveillance. For example, Lou was marathon training, and her posts were being monitored by a friend's boyfriend through her friend's Instagram account, as discussed in her final interview:

> 'It was quite funny, a friend of mine; her boyfriend was also training and basically, he was using my Instagram posts through her to work out if he was on track or not. I'd constantly get "oh Kev was asking how far you'd run this week. I showed him your post. It was 18 miles". I was worried that someone else is using me as a guide, I'm like "stick to your own plan, I don't know what I'm doing, I'm just following a different plan" (...) I think I had one week where I dropped down to a 10-mile run, and she said "he's asked why, he looks really worried". I was like "no, no, no. My plan just had a slightly lower distance this week to then build up next week. I think it's just to give your body a break," and she was like now "he thinks his plan is wrong" and I was like "no, tell him not to stress. Tell him I was being lazy."' (Lou, final interview, 29, F)

In this instance, intriguingly, the individual who was also marathon training was using his girlfriend's Instagram account (a close friend of Lou's) to view and track Lou's posts. This was not purely for the purpose of surveillance but to use Lou's training schedule and progress as a guide for his own development. As Lou described when she tapered her runs, her friend's boyfriend was worried his training plan was 'wrong' as he considered Lou a demonstration of expertise. In turn, Lou felt she had to legitimate her shorter run, describing it as 'lazy' to her friend, so her boyfriend did not feel anxious that his training plan was incorrect or that he was incompetent. This interaction demonstrates how once the participants' posts were shared on social media, surveillance from others extended further than their online community, into their online communities' social network, both online and offline. In this instance, Lou's friend's boyfriend, who did not 'follow' Lou on Instagram, surveyed her posts through his girlfriend's account. Surveillance, therefore, through these posts is indeterminable and not bounded within online networks or the individuals we choose to 'follow' or 'friend' us.

Participants acknowledged that knowing individuals within and outside of their online community were using their posts as a guide and tool for their own training practices became a real pressure. Being aware of this, they then felt they had to undertake certain practices and to document them for the now-known extended community's gaze. As Lou stated:

> 'It did become a self-perpetuating thing of like actually now do I need to do that so, he feels that he's on track or because of that lower week, I'm a few miles behind every week. Is that going to make him feel better? That sort of became a bit too much (...). Just do what you're doing.' (Lou, final interview, 29, F)

Once she knew her friend's boyfriend was using her as a training guide, Lou felt compelled to keep tracking and sharing her runs for his benefit to ensure he could track himself against her. She also ensured she included context in her posts to let others know where she was in her training plan. For example, in Figure 3.1 she details that after a 20 mile run she will now be 'tapering' to give her body a break, before the marathon in a few weeks' time.

Simultaneously, this level of accountability to these now-known and imagined communities was no longer simply a motivator for Lou but a pressure to be the guide and motivator for others watching. Therefore, for fear of negative community comparison and competition, participants adopted more extreme or intense exercise behaviours (Goodyear et al, 2017: 8). Lou personalised her posts to provide context for her personalised targets, with the hope that the community would similarly personalise their own training plans. She also tried to distance her sense of responsibility towards the viewing community by individualising her posts. These pressures, when prolonged over months of marathon training, felt distracting; not only did she find it hard to simply focus on her own training plan and personal goals but her concern was that she now knew the community would similarly be finding her posts both motivating and distracting. Participants stated that being used as a training guide, or role model (as identified throughout the research findings), made it challenging to focus on themselves, as they were consistently concerned with how others were perceiving them. Perhaps this is the eternal paradox of sharing 'health' and fitness-related content (or any content arguably) on social media.

Figure 3.1: Lou's 'tapering run'

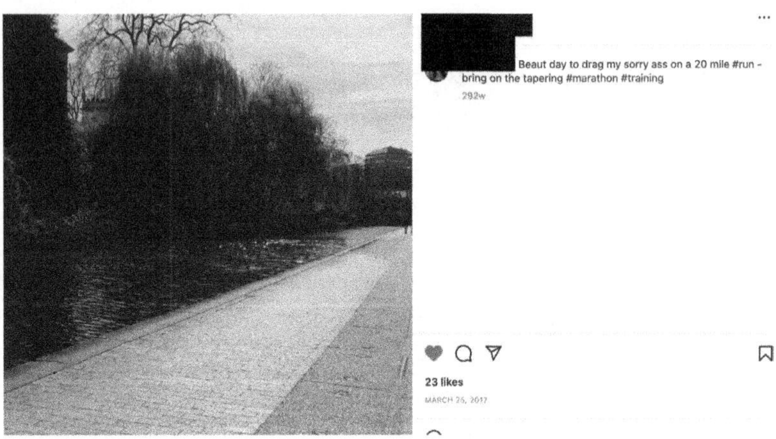
Beaut day to drag my sorry ass on a 20 mile #run - bring on the tapering #marathon #training
292w
23 likes
MARCH 25, 2017

Gratification is felt when positive feedback is received from the community, which motivates further 'healthy' practices and sharing, but over time, being the object of others' gaze creates pressures, which can distract the user from personal goals and personal gratification. These findings chime with Ruckenstein and Pantzar's (2017: 410) analysis, which identifies how through 'feedback loops, people are approached as computer-like information processors, or "auto-correlating servomechanisms," a living part of a dataistic apparatus that allows the reflection and regulation of specific movements and behaviour'. These surveillant assemblages similarly evolve into competitive and comparative practices, which regularly operate in a challenging and derogative way through public insults from others. The presentation of data and exercise is used directly as a competitive tool against others within the online community. However, amidst attempts to undermine other self-trackers within these social networks, negative feedback from and fierce competition with other users were at times interpreted as being a source of advice and support, for which one should not feel apologetic or sensitive. Roy expressed that within the community when he saw someone giving wrong advice to another weightlifter he felt frustrated as he self-proclaimed that he was a better teacher:

> 'I'm very unapologetic when I'm criticising someone.' (Roy, first interview, 26, M)

> His girlfriend is an excellent lifter but has never really taught anything. I on the other hand have been tutoring/teaching/helping people learn for almost 8 years. This is a pretty common theme in the fitness world, where people assume just that because someone is successful, it means they can teach (…) but it's not a qualification in and of itself (…) it frustrates me that his basics are probably going to be off, because he's starting off on the wrong foot, with a level of complexity unconducive to learning. (Roy, diary entry, 26, M)

Roy highlights an interesting contradiction here, with regard to demonstrating expertise by sharing online, in that it does not necessarily translate into having any related qualification. Who has the qualifications to call themselves an expert online? Here the murky division of roles between layperson, expert, professional, teacher, nutritionist, medic and even doctor becomes blurred, through the use of self-tracking apps and social media. The ambiguity of these devices, which act as both medical and consumer monitors, even though their validity has not been scientifically proven, combined with the context collapse of audiences and members on Facebook and Instagram, further destabilises the idea of voices of authority (Buyx and Prainsack, 2012). Before these devices entered mainstream consumerism, medics held the professional authority and expertise of biometric analysis through access to technology, training and qualifications. The question can therefore be asked as to whether a hierarchy should exist within these hybrid 'health' and wellness devices, in terms of users, roles and representations of health, fitness and the body. As Ziebland and Wyke (2012: 234) assert: 'Learning through other people's experiences may sometimes prevent unnecessary consultations.' Here Ziebland and Wyke discuss patients sharing online, but the same surveillance and guiding practices are identifiable when participants train towards specific 'health' and fitness goals. For example, in Lou's case, she had previously run marathons but felt concerned that other marathon runners were using her posts as a training guide when she was not a professional runner. In contrast, Roy had taught before and felt frustrated that when seeing others teaching with poor or incorrect instructions it made him feel competitive within his online community with regard to 'who "gets to be his teacher"' (Roy, diary entry, 26, M).

Giving 'advice' and being 'supportive', as the user interprets it, can, however, turn users against one another. Nevertheless, this does not alter the overall interactions and dynamics within the community, as users tend to continue sharing, feeding back or trolling one another. However, a lot of 'genuine' support is gained through seemingly healthy competition and one-to-one feedback. For Jennie, the online community explicitly told her she would need their support. This narrative of self-betterment, of moving from one state ('unhealthy') to another ('healthy'), was frequently presented as achievable only when receiving community support. For many sharers, self-achievement and personal gratification were reinforced through the supportive gaze of the community. Particularly for those who do not have 'offline' or 'real friends' undertaking these health transformations, the audience feedback online aids their supposed development.

Unwelcome participation and feedback are sometimes received from these audiences. Amy (first interview, 27, F) was regularly posting Facebook status updates, documenting her cancer diagnosis and health journey. On one occasion, she was crowdfunding for some treatments, which were not available on the British National Health Service. She received a private Facebook message from a family 'friend', asking her who she thought she was and why she was 'so special she deserved other people's money?' (Amy, first interview, 27, F). Understandably, Amy was shocked at this negative feedback from her online community. Yet she just accepted it was someone with different views and it did not affect her future posts. This reflects Trottier's (2012) arguments related to how social media communities' interpersonal relationships have become increasingly surveillant. This normalises users' acceptance of unwelcome or negative feedback through the 'death of anonymity' (Bauman and Lyon, 2013: 21). The participants interpreted this not particularly as a problem but as a condition of participation. Similarly, Annie received some unwelcome feedback in the form of inappropriate comments on her Facebook Live videos. This referred to sexually explicit comments from Facebook users, who Annie did not know:

> I do get some, interesting comments on the morning live feed. As it's public, anyone from anywhere can log in and so I can get some inappropriate conversation. However, you must take the rough with the smooth and so I just ignore them! (Annie, diary entry, 28, F)

In the final interview, Annie detailed that she was not shocked or offended by these comments. She just considered them as an expected interaction on social media. She did not feel harassed and simply blocked these users. What was perhaps most interesting about these interactions was how users did not often express feelings of being harassed or upset when cruel and derogatory comments were made, and they simply brushed these interactions off as a 'necessary evil' of sharing within social networks. Thus, in data-sharing cultures, the question can be asked as to whether users have simply accepted that trolling, with foul, vulgar or sexist comments, is a part and parcel of these spheres. These examples demonstrate Tufecki's (2008), boyd and Hargittai's (2010) and Moore's (2017) identification of a 'trade off' occurring between managing privacy and achieving visibility in the eyes of others through these technologies. I can further extend these arguments through Bauman and Lyon's proposition that if we position ourselves as consumables, which arguably all social media users are, then 'to consume means nowadays not so much the delights of the palate, as investing in one's own social membership, which in the society of consumers translates as "saleability"' (2013: 32). Therefore, privacy is nullified to gain public exposure, and derogatory or negative feedback is not criticised but normalised as a part of data-sharing processes and cultures.

Being perceived as 'healthy' and 'active' by the social media community is important to users' sense of self and health identity. Community members feeding back positively to participants' posts in the form of 'likes' and written affirmations made them feel proud, not only about their own practices and sharing but also about their ability to 'inspire' others. Seeing other online friends' posts encouraged them to look forward to offline interactions and sociality:

> It's quite habitual to use if I check it. I'm going to Berlin in April with a lot of people I follow on IG [Instagram], so every time I see a post by one of them, I look forward to it more. (Roy, diary entry, 26, M)

Roy is a member of a Facebook group and community of hand-balancers and weightlifters. The members of this community mostly document their progress by posting photos and videos on their Facebook group and having (offline) meets every few months. For Roy and the other participants who are members of fitness communities, seeing other community members posting certain developments encourages them to similarly want to develop their own skills. It also adds to feelings of community, communal development and personal skill. If one member is advancing well, Roy highlighted that he would particularly look forward to meeting this individual to train and develop their skills together. The connection between community and the understanding of others doing similar practices provided comfort and can be seen as a supportive tool in this motivating discourse of self-betterment. Sophie similarly reiterated this discourse when she stated: 'It encourages me to be healthier the more I post' (Sophie, first interview, 31, F).

In response to such community surveillance, a reflexive process ensues. The more these users self-track, share and reflect on these practices with the community, the 'healthier' they feel. The process of reflexivity is a motivating and guiding tool to maintain 'healthy' practices, whereby lifestyle is strategically managed through the surveillant practices in the liquid surveillant and digital society (Lyon and Bauman, 2013).

Input versus output health management discourse

Such management of health through surveillance for self-trackers also develops through what I term an input versus output discourse. As this chapter has explored, the process of self-surveillance and self-tracking seeks to tell us something about our bodies and encourages 'health optimisation' (Wolf, 2010). As Waltz (2012: 4) asserts: 'seeing our own biological data in front of us (…) can affect our behaviour.' This was a common interpretation amongst self-trackers, who perceived bodily health as an entity that needed to be individually 'managed' through the instrumentalisation of a controlling and powerful mind and technology (Moore and Robinson, 2016). In this process, the mechanical workings of the body become reduced to a negotiation between inputs and outputs (Gregory, 2013). Such conceptualisations of the body as modifiable and interpretable through objective mechanisation reflect scientific ideals stemming from the nineteenth century, which reduced human interpretation to mechanical evidence (Daston and Galison, 2010; Kristensen and Ruckenstein, 2018). The idea that human 'enlightenments' can be obtained only by 'objective machines' similarly reflects data utopian discourses, which promote the perspective that better health is achievable only by self-monitoring through self-tracking data. However, this is possible only if you have the willingness and self-discipline to respond to and act upon such information.

Self-trackers often conceptualised their bodies as engines or machines. In essence, what you put in, you will get out. This becomes interpreted as re-addressing the balance of 'health' through individual self-disciplinary behaviours. This discourse suggests and supports the argument that self-surveillance and tracking will transform and revolutionise healthcare (Bottles, 2012; Moore and Robinson, 2016; Moore, 2017). As Wolf (2010: np) suggests: 'numbers [which they are tracking] hold secrets that they can't afford to ignore, including answers to questions they have not yet thought to ask.' The user can subjectively decipher the objective nature of statistical self-quantification and tracking, as no finite goal is outlined. Beato (2012) argues that 'self-trackers' monitor to increase control over their own lives.

There is a paucity of literature that addresses the reality of these claims by examining the process undertaken by users. This book examines this gap and identifies that the accumulation and examination of data create extreme self-regulating pressures for self-trackers, thus provoking stress and anxiety. As Purpura (2011: 7) asserts, these anxieties can occur 'by pulling quantitative measures to the foreground over qualitative ones and usurping the normal situational human decision-making process'. This dissolves the division between the interior and exterior of the body and blurs the distinctions between the biological, the social (Rose, 2013) and the technological. Purpura et al (2011: 7) highlight how these 'borderlines between encouragement, persuasion, and coercion, and specifically with who should be in control of individual behaviour [are blurred]. Persuasive computing (...) participates in and reinforces broader troublesome cultural trends to control the body.' The users are presented with a cultural construction and 'datafication' of their biometrics over a physical construction of their bodies. This individualised, internalised and self-policing discourse pertains that healthy behaviours is best enabled through a continual cycle of self-management and self-care. Whether the information provided tells the user anything 'new' or indeed helpful at all is open to question. These practices reduce 'human experience to inputs and outputs [and] raises the questions: am I man or machine?' (Purpura et al, 2011: 6). Furthermore, another question can be asked: How do I negotiate between my human interpretation of experience and mechanical evidence of my experience? As this user recognised, 'It is interesting that something has forced me to take that look on my life' (Lara, first interview, 28, F).

This 'forced' recognition within self-tracking devices ensures that capturing and sharing data are based upon what the device deems to fall within categories of importance, in this case food, drink and exercise. Lara's account reminds us that data is not neutral, as it is selective about what is and is not captured. As Duffy (2014: np) asserts: 'data scientists are storytellers, interpreters. They take slices of information from the data-sphere around us and translate them into something for us to consume.' The 'meaning' making from the data visualised extends further than Duffy (2014) proposes here. In fact, rather than providing something for the user to consume (and then share), the visualisations are inductive and enable the creation of a data story that 'shape[s] assumptions and promises of visibility and knowing, further connecting to research on how digital devices and the data that they generate configure knowledge spaces in society' (Ruckenstein, 2017: 84). As acknowledged by Jennie (first interview, 40, F): 'It gives you the visual reminders and cues for staying on track.'

This spreadsheet input versus output approach to managing health is problematic and oversimplifies the complexities of the human body, whereby design prompts directly impact 'health' practices, reflecting Moore's (2017: np) argument that 'machines are tools of quantification and division, compartmentalisation and potentially control'. This is particularly applicable to the area of human instinct. For example, when a running application prompts a user who is feeling unwell to go for a run (and there is no way to 'track' or 'monitor' a flu or common cold), physical exertion might make the user more unwell, but the device nudges them to go. Therefore, the question remains: Who do you listen to, your disciplinary exercise regime, your device or platform, or your body? These practices perceive the plasticity of the body and brain as malleable, through calculated forms of intervention, for example exercise or eating 'healthily'. This malleable approach to the body and 'health' management ensures the presentation of calculated interventions (health and wellness apps, platforms and lifestyle advice), which promote health as an entity to be individually tailored and self-managed. Take the following example of Tim, which demonstrates that his work commitments have a big impact on the leisure and free time available in which to exercise or prepare healthy meals. Many self-trackers maintain that the availability (or lack) of free and leisure time outside of work is a key factor in enabling or preventing 'healthy' decisions and lifestyles. Tim is a keen yogi and posted daily about his practice and development. With his focus on yoga and constant sharing of his practice, there was not much time left for preparing 'healthy' meals:

> 'Pretty much every Thursday after yoga class me and Jake go and get a kebab on the way home. It's because there's a very nice kebab shop next to where that is and you can justify it to yourself. I would feel bad, (…) if I didn't exercise so much. If I didn't do lots of yoga or go to the gym then my diet would actually be better than it is now. I think sometimes I almost sacrifice eating well to exercise more (…) If I don't exercise on a certain night, that's the night I tend to eat the best because I've got the time to do it.' (Tim, final interview, 34, M)

Tim frequently sacrificed making, in his own words, 'healthy' nutritious food so he could exercise instead, because he felt food shopping and meal preparation were too 'time consuming'. He acknowledged that because he exercised daily, he was not overly concerned that he was not eating 'well'. Time spent at the gym and practicing yoga, to enable the documentation of his fitness and skill development on social media, became the priority, rather than buying, preparing and enjoying fresh, 'healthy' homemade food. Because Tim did not consider himself a 'foodie' or enjoy cooking, the expertise and 'health' status he wanted to represent online was of his fitness ability. Therefore, his leisure time was spent prioritising this over focusing upon eating 'healthy' food. Tim presented himself online as a fit, able and experienced yogi, which became his dominant 'health' identity and provided the discursive underpinnings of his posting: prioritising good 'health' as physical fitness and demonstration of yogic practice over the nutrition he put in his body to fuel these physically intense behaviours and commitments. Tim was sacrificing 'healthy' food to exercise more, and indeed it is important to critique and question how (un)healthy this actually is.

Prioritisation of time is an interesting aspect here for the user, in terms of the allocation of time for and justification of various tasks (exercise versus rest, or exercise versus preparing 'healthy' food). Such a balancing act demonstrates challenging health contentions for these individuals in their everyday lives. These input versus output discourses, which present management of the body like a machine (Purpura et al, 2011), prioritise intervention through prevention or rectification (Moore and Robinson, 2016; Moore, 2017). These strategies of intervention cultivate a habit of precaution, prevention and pre-emption, whereby health can be 'maintained' and improved by prioritising some 'healthy' behaviours, such as exercising, over others. For example, consuming junk food or alcohol could be rectified by enacting 'healthy' behaviours once again. A lack of response to device information or nudges, and a general lack of self-surveillance, means that the individual management of 'health' may fail because of a lack of monitored intervention. One of the reflexive diary questions asked participants what, if anything, influenced their health decisions. Frequently, users answered that by managing 'healthy' decisions the following day they felt they could 'rectify' earlier poor 'health' management, demonstrating the dominant proliferation of the input versus output quantification discourse surrounding health optimisation (Gregory, 2013) This was demonstrated by Tim's love of 'junk' or 'unhealthy' foods, which he felt he could 'work off' in the gym:

> What I was eating at the time was mostly influenced by what was available nearby and what I had time to eat/prepare. Which was

> mostly Greggs and takeaways (…) time to purchase and prepare food at this time was so small I caved in and went with the easy options. I did however exercise extra hard this night in an attempt to burn off those extra calories from all the junk food!! (Tim, diary entry, 34, M)

Many of the users ate 'convenient' foods but legitimated and accepted this because they could work off the calories in the gym and not focus on, or avoid, the fact that they were not eating nutritious foods. They recognised that exercising meant they did not feel guilty about eating 'unhealthy' foods or consuming alcohol. Furthermore, certain 'unhealthy' or carb-heavy foods have to be made 'legitimate' to eat not just for pleasure' but for a 'cheat day'. On further questioning this practice in her final interview, Sophie explained that her 'cheat day' legitimates pasta (recognised as a 'bad' carb-heavy lunch), but she then excuses this 'cheat' by saying that it will help fuel and therefore aid her run:

> I ate the pasta because I was going for the run. I wouldn't eat pasta on a non-cheat day, so it worked out well. (Sophie, diary entry, 31, F)

> Had a good run, did feel able to go out later on without feeling guilty about eating/ drinking later on. (Lou, diary entry, 29, F)

> Today was a full rest/cheat day for sure! Motivated by weeks of being active, eating reasonably well so I figured I deserved a lazy day! (Tim, diary entry, 34, M)

Interestingly, the dominant narrative of 'rest days' enabled participants to have guilt and shame free 'lazy' days to balance 'active' and healthy days. Through extended self-surveying practices to maintain self-regulation and 'healthy' behaviours, overall the participants felt productive by managing their 'health' to enable self-improvement and the propagation of 'healthier' bodies, which was positively interpreted. Annie interpreted these positive feelings as feeling better through eating well and feeling 'good' about adhering to self-proclaimed goals around diet:

> I've been quite good with my food, and it definitely does make me feel better… I find eating rubbish makes you feel 'greasy'… I don't like feeling greasy! ☺ (Annie, diary entry, 28, F).

The overall discourse illustrated by the users, however, was that eating badly or not exercising can be rectified and 'overcome' by exercising harder, minimising calories or eating 'healthier' nutritious food, regardless of what one has previously put into their bodies. Self-trackers perceived the pre-emption of the 'negative' effects of unhealthy behaviours or consumption to be rectified by intervention via 'healthy' practices. When thinking about the temporal nature of the practices subsequently adopted through poor 'health' management or behaviours, the dominant discourse advocates that the poor choices surrounding 'health' can be immediately overcome by an instantaneous lifestyle overhaul and 'personal rehabilitation' (Cederstrom and Spicer, 2015: 134). Regardless of the way lifestyle behaviours may have been in the past, and whether they can be rectified, the body and 'health' can be immediately transformed into a 'healthy' subject through self-surveillance, regulation and self-discipline. This discourse advocates that the body works like a machine that harnesses an input versus output engine, which suggests that if you eat 'unhealthy' food or drink (input) you can rectify the extra calories by burning this off (output).

Conclusions

There is a dynamic function creep of surveillance practices for self-trackers. Surveillance is used for self-monitoring as well as for peer and imagined surveillance within social media environments, with the seductive nature of these devices and technologies for users being the promise of connectivity as well as health optimisation, community support and appreciation. However, as many of these platforms and applications are free to use, users freely give up personal data, which is often unknowingly mined by the service providers and third parties (Zuboff, 2019). This data is frequently perceived by users as the ideological and practical 'trade-off' for using the 'free' service. Participants in this research frequently viewed peer surveillance and data mining not as an invasion of their privacy but rather as an acceptable practice that is an intricate part of daily use of these technologies. Furthermore, community and peer surveillance were perceived and enacted as an accountability and motivating tool for many self-trackers. Whether you perceive this as useful or empowering, or exploitative and privacy invading, there is an undeniable accepted asymmetry in power between those who collect and mine data and those from whom it is collected (Andrejevic, 2013). This asymmetric power is accompanied by an asymmetric transparency. Whether they know it or not, users are increasingly the subjects of dataveillance (van Dijck, 2014), a totalising process of surveillance through the many and ubiquitous points of access in our digital society.

Users cannot negotiate their privacy rights, which means that surveillance and visibility, therefore, become an integral and accepted practice of interpersonal relations within self-tracking technologies and social media communities, as users accept how their personal data is a form of lucrative surveillance. Surveillance, on and via these platforms, operates in more obscure and omnipresent ways; when the body is used as a site for surveillance via use of these technologies, we normalise and even reinforce the bio-politics of our human existence, which is enacted through and operates on three levels within practices of 'governmentality': individual, technological and state. I argue that the state, the technology and the individual user are all agents of power, co-evolving together through practices of overt and covert surveillance. Illustrated using the surveillant stages and practices examined throughout this chapter, of self-trackers' ambiguous health goals of self-betterment, their pride in self-surveillance, whilst navigating the power imbalances of agential boundaries with using technology to manage health. In turn, this leads to a competition with one's own body *and* device, sometimes through expected community surveillance online, and often through the mechanical reductions of the body that these devices and platforms enable. Therefore, I do not conceive of co-evolving as a utopian growth but an ever pervasive and subtle regulatory one. In new materialist terms, the mind with technology is conceived as a powerful domain and tool to increasingly control the malleable body due to socio-economic and political ideology, whereby, citizens are continually subjected to normalising regimes of regulatory surveillance, and with it, associated reductive and oversimplifying notions of what is and is not health, wellness or fitness improvements.

4

Discipline and Moralism of Our Health

This chapter examines 'health' fitness and lifestyle management in relation to neoliberal moral self-disciplinary discourses, which position the human being and body as a subject to be worked upon. This neoliberal ideology stemmed from a distancing from state interventions, through the promotion of the idea that individuals have a responsibility towards wider institutional, systemic and capitalist systems of control, which situate the 'indebted man' as the subjective figure of contemporary capitalism (Lazzarato, 2006). The 'indebted' population, therefore, is a paradoxical structure of neoliberal societies, whereby debt must be fulfilled in order to be 'free'. As Rose (2007: 90) asserts: 'subjects obliged to be free were required to conduct themselves responsibly to account for their own lives.' The moral dimensions within dominant 'health' discourses have become inherent within current self-surveillance practices (as discussed in Chapter 3) and the regulatory design of self-tracking apps, devices and the sharing of related content on social media. Within discourses of self-tracking and 'bad' health, self-worth can become tied to data (Carmichael, 2010). This chapter critiques these discourses, to examine the problematic and moral issues that arise from adhering to such regulatory practices. This book draws upon the definition of moralisation as proposed by Paul Rozin (2011: 380), as 'the acquisition of moral qualities by objects and activities that were previously morally neutral'. These 'health' surveillance and tracking practices intrinsically assign an individual moral obligation to preserve one's own health as public duty, free from state or institutional support (Knowles, 1997: 64). This discourse of 'shame' and guilt was identifiable throughout this research project's empirical data, embodied in relation to 'bad' and 'unhealthy' decisions. This chapter examines the (perceived) lack of self-discipline, health anxieties that legitimate inactivity, self-surveillance and the moralism of body image and, lastly, the burden of self-surveillance and self-tracking as some of the key moralising and regulatory practices of the digital health self today.

Identifying the moralism and disciplining of health

The moralism of health is not a new discourse in healthcare communication. It can be traced back to the seventeenth century, when religious discourses associated poor health with sinful behaviour (Mennel et al, 1992; Brandt and Rozin, 1997). This archaic perspective positions poor health as being a result of sinful behaviour and therefore as something to be individually shameful for (Mennel et al, 1992; Brandt and Rozin, 1997). In Chapter 1, I established how this discourse still exists today through a detailed analysis of the socio-economic, cultural and political shifts post-World War Two until the current day and COVID-19 pandemic. Medicine has historically been presented as being objective, 'configured as the antithesis of the world of morals. Medicine is scientific, objective and definite – morals are subjective, relative and indeterminate (…) often viewed as a source of stigma and despair for patients' (Brandt and Rozin, 1997: 7). The blurring of health with morality still exists pervasively today, and the discourse is reflected throughout media, press and public health messaging and social media narratives and illustrated extensively in the empirical data from this research project.

If we follow Foucault's (1986) definitions of morality as a process of ethical self-stylisation through care of the self, the 'moral self' can be understood and related to through validation of being 'good enough' in its 'health'-related behaviours. In this regard, the individual moralism of 'health' is, to a point, relative to what individuals subjectively decide are their own regulatory barriers and rules, in line with wider socio-cultural norms of healthy behaviours and bodies presented by social and mass media. For, as Metzl (2010: 3) highlights:

> Calling such language sexism or cultural narcissism would mobilize a particular critique. But calling it 'health' allows (…) [the ability] to seamlessly construct certain bodies as desirable whilst relegating others as obscene. The result explicitly justifies particular corporeal types and practices while implicitly suggesting that those who do not play along suffer from ill health.

Therefore, the 'health' moralism discourse operates through an internalisation of shame, in turn encouraging self-regulatory and self-disciplinary 'health' behaviours. This reinforces how the morals and values ascribed to 'health' and 'illness' are fluid, and constructed socio-culturally, rather than existing as physical concepts or states of being (King and Watson, 2005: 37). With the neoliberal focus on lower healthcare costs, higher risks become associated with higher costs and their moral consequences, thereby linking health risks with individual moral decision-making (Cederstrom and Spicer, 2015) and its detrimental impact on population health. As Buyx and Prainsack (2012: 81) assert:

> If we feel pressured by our social and political environment to undertake every possible preventative and predictive measure to learn about and decrease the existing risks, and if we invest more time and effort in this, we may feel a grudge against those who spend their time and money in more pleasurable ways, and who therefore, we think, incur additional risks (read: costs).

This perspective is problematic as it assigns degrees of risk based upon individual lifestyle choices, which assumes direct causal links between the two. This is not a satisfactory explanation, as it is sometimes impossible to prove why a particular condition affected an individual (Buyx and Prainsack, 2012). For example, as Chapter 2 identified, the choice architecture and regulatory design tools of these applications and devices 'nudge' and prompt users to make certain 'health' choices (such as lower calorie consumption) and to undertake certain health behaviours (such as exercising or running further). Purpura et al (2011) argue that the functions of these applications must be recognised as powerful regulatory tools, arguably coercing users to undertake certain actions that cannot be individually tailored to each user and may inflict damaging physical pressure upon the body as well as additional psychological pressure on the minds of the users. So, individuals integrating health technology and social media into their everyday lives, as health management tools or for guidance, use technology as a technique to help adjust or confine 'health'-related decision-making processes within the parameters of perceived morally 'right' consumption choices, articulated through data collection, representation and interpretation (Fajans, 2013). This involvement positions the citizen as a consumer who actively makes the 'right' ethical decision for the management of their health and self-care. Self-regulation, therefore, can be identified as a heightened monitoring of self-surveillance, whereby this regulation may or may not impact upon behaviours but may become modified in line with adhering to 'healthy' discourses, which influence the participants' sense of moral self as 'good' or 'bad', 'healthy' or 'unhealthy', individuals.

Self-discipline can therefore be understood as a type of self-regulation and a step towards self-policing. Self-policing directly impacts upon and influences individual 'health' and fitness-related practices and behaviours. Self-discipline, then, is the adherence to rules and self-regulations advocated through societal discourses surrounding the moralism of 'health'. Furthermore, this dictates behaviour modifications in relation to what makes a 'healthy' or 'healthier' individual, in whatever capacity it is subjectively determined or interpreted. Of course, subjectivity must be recognised within these decision-making processes. However, this chapter situates these practices of self-surveillance, regulation and discipline within wider neoliberal socio-economic, cultural and political discourses of individualised responsibility towards self-care. This was demonstrated throughout the research findings, as the positive feelings users initially associated with self-tracking and the governance of health and self-care dissipated over time and were replaced by feelings of pressure and stress. For example, the practices of quantifying and tracking food and calorie intake through calorie counting apps such as MyFitnessPal can over time become 'obsessive' and a cause of anxiety for many users:

> I was actually using My Fitness Pal app previously to track my calories and macros. From today I've decided to stop using it as it has become too obsessive. I've literally spent hours before on it lying in bed at night deciding what I am allowed to eat the next day and stressing when the macros didn't add up. I can now see feeling guilty because I was only allowed 1 apple and actually had like 2 and it's messed up my carbs and sugar intake goal for the day is ridiculous. (Sophie, diary entry, 31, F)

These self-tracking and self-quantification processes over extended periods of time felt over-regulatory and an embodiment of self-disciplinary rules and quantifications of consumption, exercise, routine and, broadly, lifestyle. Here we see how 'individual strivings for health, are, in some circumstances, rendered more difficult by the ways in which health is cultural configured and socially sustained (…) health is a concept, a norm, and a set of bodily practices whose ideological work is often rendered invisible by the assumption that is it a monolithic, universal good' (Metzl, 2010: 9). How this translates into ambiguities leads towards 'ridiculous' determinants of what users considered they were and were not allowed to do and eat, which they interpreted as impacting upon their sense of self-worth, generating feelings of being a 'bad' and immoral person. Shame and guilt were attached to poor self-discipline and not sticking to self-imposed 'rules'. Furthermore, feelings of elation and control became synonymous with an adherence to self-imposed individual parameters. Although at both ends of these 'good' and 'bad' spectrums users acknowledged that extreme or overwhelming feelings in relation to perceived success or moral failure as a result of self-surveillance, regulation and discipline were 'silly', self-indulgent and 'foolish', they still held regulatory and moral ruling over how they perceived themselves.

(Perceived) lack of self-discipline

Perceptions of poor self-discipline, a lack of self-surveillance and not maintaining 'healthy' behaviours prompted emotionally embodied embarrassment and guilt for many users. Matt, a weightlifter and gymnast, suffered an injury and spoke frequently about his frustrations of 'slipping out' of 'normal routines'.

Users often identify how changing eating habits and consuming 'unhealthy' snack foods manifested itself as feelings of guilt and that they 'should' be self-disciplining regardless of injury. This is particularly prevalent over celebratory or holiday periods such as Christmas; 'I found myself thinking I can't believe I ate that much; you give yourself a hard time. I'm constantly obsessed' (Sophie, diary entry, 31, F). Failure to 'actively' maintain 'health' engenders guilt for the individual where previously there may have been very little. Robert Frank (1988) argued that one key function of emotions is to keep us on a biologically and culturally adaptive track, like love reducing infidelity, for example. Therefore,

> a number of emotions can be thought of in the service of socialisation, and hence vehicles for relating morality to behaviours and preferences. Unpleasant emotions such as embarrassment, shame, guilt, and disgust direct behaviour by causing us to cease doing things that have already aroused them. These emotions are elicited by primarily situations dictated by our socialisation experience. (Rozin, 1997: 384)

Gregory (2013: 8) asserts that self-tracking technologies may have damaging qualities, created through the 'sense of guilt they engender implying defeat when users go "over" their allotted calories and then recommending exercise to make it up', which was reflected throughout the user accounts from this empirical data. This had a large impact on how individuals conduct their everyday lives and interpersonal relationships online and offline. For many users, being seen to eat unhealthily, however, infrequently generated particular embarrassment, especially when offline practices did not match online representations of a healthy lifestyle:

> 'I tell you what, Friday and Saturday night I had McDonalds, and a new girl moved into the house (…) I felt mortified that she saw me eat McDonalds two nights in a row. I was obsessing over it. She thinks that's what I eat. I felt disgusting. She thinks I'm not healthy.' (Sophie, final interview, 31, F)

For many users, someone seeing them consume 'junk food', even if no opinion over these food choices was expressed, can lead them to imagine and assume others' negative judgements of their 'bad' and unhealthy choices. In turn, this can lead to a destructive internal monologue, whereby narratives of mortification and self-punishment exist; 'disgust is a powerful tool for negative socialisation; a very effective way to get people to avoid something and to have this avoidance internalised is to make the entity disgusting' (Rozin, 1997: 384). Perhaps most interestingly, and worryingly, users acknowledge that although they felt this way, they also felt they had little control over or ability to stop or 'let go' of these disciplinary surveillant practices and associated feelings of disgust:

> 'Yeah, I always feel like I'm never doing enough (…) there is this underlying thing that I'm not good enough or that I could be doing "better", or I could be "better" at everything. Maybe it's that that transpires in my running or [feeling like I am] not doing enough for my health. I always take the "oh I'm just going to rest tonight."' (Lara, final interview, 28, F)

The prevalence of this internal discourse should not be understated under neoliberal digital capitalism, which advocates that users could 'always be doing more' and makes them feel like their efforts are never 'good enough'. Overcoming mental or physical obstacles becomes a real priority for the digital health self, usually enacted to seek self-validation to feel 'good enough'. As Cederstrom and Spicer (2015: 5) argue, wellness is not a choice but a 'moral obligation', and the same can be said of health management. Those individuals who do not take up these technologies, therefore, may be 'constructed as failing to achieve this ideal and as consequently at fault for becoming ill or contracting a disease' (Lupton, 2012b: 240). This demonstrates how many self-tracking users perceive their health behaviours as reflective of morality. If they do not overcome the health-related hurdle and do not 'push themselves' to start exercising again, they consider themselves to be 'having a crisis'.

> 'Actually, there were a couple of weeks when I first moved here that I didn't train as much and that sort of led to a crisis where I didn't do a handstand for two weeks and I'm like "am I just going to stop?"' (Roy, final interview, 26, M)

Not maintaining healthy behaviours, such as going to the gym, prompts questions of users' commitment to their regimes and to their health, which was at times a form of personal torment. This moralisation of 'health' ensured that the participants sought validation from themselves in the context of these post-modern self-reflexive times (Giddens, 1991). In this vision, attempts at maintaining 'self-discipline' and being morally 'good' are continually at the fore, although they are not always acted upon, and are a cause of ongoing angst. Therefore, regulation through self-surveying practices in the process of self-tracking parallels 'broader shifts in identity construction, [whereby] people are no longer bound to the inherited guidelines of the past, morality becomes a project to be worked out, designed and depicted in relation to others' (Hookway and Graham, 2017: np). In this way, the moralism of health is arguably inherent in post-modern reflexive practices and is constructed and enacted upon through self-tracking and social media management and performativity of 'health'.

Being perceived as morally 'good enough' must often fall in line with specified regulatory frameworks set by the users, for example, exercising on certain days or eating 'healthily' six days a week. Furthermore, when this activity is reduced to tracking, graphs or numbers it does not respect the user's 'self-esteem' (Wolf, 2010). As Wolf (2010: np) asserts: 'Electronic trackers have no feelings. The objectivity of a machine can [either] seem generous or merciless, tolerant or cruel.' This moralised datafication of 'health' through the measurement of such regulation, either internally or through capture on self-tracking devices, enables subjectively determined 'legitimate' times of renounced moral 'codes' and rules, for example, 'cheat days' (indulge in 'unhealthy' foods) or 'rest days' (not exercising). This similarly reflects and reinforces input versus output discourses with regard to 'health' management, whereby poor 'health' practices can be overcome by enacting 'healthy' behaviours and similarly 'healthy' behaviours can be undone by 'unhealthy' consumption or not exercising. This was reflected in Lara's diary entry:

> [I] had a couple of quite boozy nights so was a bit worried about getting my ass back in gear with running and not being a hungover mess for the weekend and getting my focus back. (Lara, diary entry, 28, F)

Behaving rationally and returning to regulation according to subjectively defined rules mean renouncing the interdictions required to remove or prevent 'bad' and 'unhealthy' behaviours. Here we can identify, in the context of public health discourses and practices, a shift from a centralised disciplinary control society towards multiple delineated and disciplinary societies and individuals (Rose, 1999). These fragmented and adopted practices arise through a complex embodiment of citizenship responsibilities and self-management of the body. As Ajana (2005: 3) succinctly explains: 'Discipline and control are interwoven within the fabric of everyday interactions.' These regulations encourage external pressures to become internally assimilated by these users through an individual moralism of 'health', whereby following such regulations advocated 'good' and 'healthy' behaviours and resistance to or an active choice to disavow the 'nudges' manifested itself in individualised conceptualisations of immorality and the associated dimensions of guilt, shame and embarrassment. Each individual is made responsible for a new ethics of self-management, obliged to take responsibility for their own 'health', not just to identify and manage their susceptibilities but to optimise themselves through diet, exercise, supplements and health knowledge.

Furthermore, as Cederstrom and Spicer (2015: 49) argue, guilt can be seductive and plays an important role in commanding the self 'to be healthy (…) with a not-so-subtle underlying message: If you don't shackle yourself to a diet, carefully monitor your weight and seek to get back to some kind of imagined original state (…) then you are a morally defiled person.' A desire to be 'healthy' and to prolong our lives binds us to 'health' and to 'experts' or 'influencers' who, whether qualified or not, patent new lifestyles, diets and risks, leaving every aspect of the life course vulnerable to commercial exploitation in the name of 'health' (Rose, 2007). Take, for example, teen self-trackers: between 67 per cent and 92 per cent of teens report using social media for health information (fitness, sexual health and nutrition), but many of them are unable to identify reliable health information and most will use social media over National Health Service, Public Health England and the Department of Health (Plaisime et al, 2020). Furthermore, research by the University of Glasgow showed that 90 per cent of the weight management advice of UK social media influencers is incorrect (Sabbagh et al, 2020). The amount of health, fitness and diet misinformation circulating online is alarming enough, without considering how reliant particularly the younger generations are upon these platforms for health guidance. As we have seen in circulation of COVID-19 misinformation, this can be detrimental to both physical and mental health. This is further analysed in our concluding chapter. In terms of the relationship between health and morality, health expertise works in alliance with individual ethics, and these modes of collaboration are hugely problematic because of their gross oversimplification of 'health' and the body. Furthermore, this alliance can have damaging implications, which occur in the form of over-exercise, misinformation or damaging one's self-esteem or mental health.

Health and fitness progression – legitimating inactivity

The frustration related to not being able to enact self-discipline and undertake 'improving' fitness practices and developments becomes an embodied pressure for self-trackers over time. Managing and mediating between long- and short-term 'health' goals can be a core strategy to legitimate not undertaking certain 'healthy' acts. In this research, inactivity or an inability to maintain 'healthy' practices for any reason, such as ill health, injury or lack of free time, was identified as frequently manifesting as feelings of stress, frustration and shame. Regardless of the reasoning behind physical inactivity or eating 'unhealthily', feelings of agitation and frustration were still prevalent. These users adhered to this neoliberal individualised responsibilisation discourse, and they felt that they 'could always be doing more'. These feelings of inadequacy and agitation frequently developed into a heightened consciousness of the self and the body. This was reflected in Matt's words:

> My lack of health and fitness activities, including nutrition, has made a massive impact upon my general mood. I'm a little more agitated and feel very frustrated with it all. (Annie, diary entry, 28, F)

> I try to be conscious of my food intake/calories, however, I've been slacking a little lately. (Matt, diary entry, 41, F)

Being 'slack' was demonstrative of poor 'health management', not instilling self-regulation and disciplinary behaviours, leading to, in Matt's case, inactivity and the over-consumption of calories. However, when this diary entry was completed, Matt was in recovery from surgery and was under strict medical instruction not to exercise. Interestingly, all the self-trackers acknowledged this real sense of 'beating oneself up' over being 'slack' despite having legitimate reasons for not engaging in certain behaviours. What is particularly interesting here is the question of why frustration was felt by the participants for not being able to do enough exercise (or burn enough calories) when an injury prevented it. Where does this pervasive embodiment of the pressure that advocates 'I should be doing more' come from, regardless of physical capabilities (or lack of)? Truth and 'evidence' are considered to be reflected in and by these devices, through what the user is doing, what the device is capturing and what the user can then share. Yet, as Purpura et al (2011: 6) highlight: 'one postulate that underlies persuasive computing is that technology is not neutral', and it most certainly does not provide truths. Rather, it presents a carefully selected 'datafication' of events and 'health'. Therefore, self-discipline in self-tracking is a mediation between what we personally want to achieve and what the application or 'persuasive computing' might tell the participant to do (Purpura et al, 2011: 6). Lara expands on this in her final interview:

> 'I think because I signed up for this race, I think there was a pressure to maintain, because I was just about up to 10 km when the doctor said I shouldn't run. I was like "I need to maintain this level because I've got this race" but then it was also like "now I've got an excuse not to do it."' (Lara, final interview, 28, F)

Interestingly, for Lara, listening to her body in pain was not an excuse not to race and such a decision had to come from a medic with an official authority to 'sign off' on her injury, which legitimated not competing in the race. Other self-trackers similarly highlighted the pressure to keep training and how pushing yourself is important to maintain progression, even if this is detrimental towards physical 'health':

> 'If I'm ill or I've had an operation, I kind of accept it but then after a few days I start to get a mixture of itchy feet in general because my body is

> used to being active and my mind is used to being pushed in that way. And a little niggle in the background is also that if I'm ill or stop doing stuff for too long then that's going to have a negative effect in terms of my slightly obsessive want for progression.' (Tim, final interview, 34, M)

What these findings illustrate is the problematic moral justification for not exercising despite being physically incapable of doing so. Furthermore, this ideological commitment to progression mentally made them feel well and 'healthy'. Even if physically able to achieve, ambiguous self-bettering or optimising goals made them feel physically 'healthier'. This demonstrates the perceived importance of mental 'health' over physical 'health', or perhaps how one informs and continually influences the other. For many users this desire for progression, fitness improvement and 'optimisation' of the self, however subjectively those goals and parameters were determined, had negative implications for their mental health, sense of self-worth and personal development. Stigma was attached to invisible ill health and injury, and the participants felt that they had to 'prove' such ailments when they were unseen, as a form of diagnostic pantomime (Roach, 2017) or representation in which the community's gaze is transported and pulled into the participants' (and patients') clinical space. It is arguable that this ties into societal anxieties associated with the mentality that body size translates as a 'moral code for everyday life, the body of the actor becomes the site of the problem. Thin or average sized people are not disciplined [or chastised] for sloth or gluttony the same way fat people are' (LeBesco, 2011: 75). For example, Tim had a hernia operation the month before participating in the research. He reflected within his diary and in the final interview that though this was an operation that resulted in a physical injury and recovery period, as it was internal, it was effectively invisible and therefore it was down to him to interpret how to 'deal' with it and decide when to exercise:

> 'I think there's a different way of conceptualising illness when it's physical, like a hernia rather than viral stuff. Legitimating illness and injury which is unseen. Yeah, you haven't got a bandage, you haven't got stitches. It's all internal, isn't it?' (Tim, final interview, 34, M)

> 'I might be feeling a bit sorry for myself and that I'm ill and weak and that I can't do it, so I probably push myself more than I should to try and change that mental state and be like "ok I can do some stuff". When I did that yoga session when I was really ill it made me feel really awful afterwards. I nearly threw up, I nearly passed out, but mentally I also felt good for it.' (Tim, final interview, 34, M)

In this quote, Tim examines how his operation was physical yet internal and thus harder to prioritise in terms of resting and recovering in the absence of the 'signs' of injury or surgery, such as stitches or bandages. Interestingly, discussing and sharing his pain and discomfort help authenticate their existence as 'pain is a motive force rarely questioned and stunning in its ability to engage us in or disengage us from the lives of other human beings' (Siebers, 2010: 183–184). Therefore, this prioritisation of rest and legitimate inactivity is made even harder when you have a viral illness, rather than a physical incapacity, which relies entirely on the individual to identify the issue for themselves. Thus, social media creates a performative sphere to 'prove' and showcase their pain and in turn legitimate a rest, recover and rejuvenation period.

Disciplinary challenges of invisible illness

Frequently in this research self-trackers failed to prevent disciplinary activities from dictating further regulatory behaviours, and they often continued to commit to these cycles of self-surveillance, regulation, and emotional strain. Without upward comparisons exemplified by others' experiences of the positive outcomes of a particular treatment or disease, people may feel increasingly distressed (Festinger, 1954). It can therefore be asked why these individuals continued with these self-imposed policing cycles of disciplinary regulation when it was detrimental to their physical and mental 'health'? Users highlighted frustrations related to being unable to exercise or eat 'healthily'. When it came to invisible disease, illness or internal injuries, they struggled to rest and let their bodies recover as they felt they would be 'losing' the physical fitness improvements they had perceivably 'gained'. Many of them pushed themselves to exercise what they considered 'healthy' physically tiresome activities, which frequently made them feel more ill but which mentally appeased them, since those activities made them feel 'productive' and able to maintain their 'healthy' lifestyle. The irony was that the attempt to 'push' oneself before being physically capable frequently delayed recovery and was at times to the detriment of their physical 'health'. In this regard, doing exercise mitigates mental anxiety, which manifests itself in a lack of activity, even if it is bad for their body. Thus, there is some tension between being 'legitimately' inactive due to rest and recovery and an inherent and embodied ambition to fulfil the objectives of 'optimisation', whereby further self-improvement becomes the desired goal for these participants. In this way, individuals strive to be 'healthy' regardless of any negative impacts upon or damage in their physical bodies.

Regulation of rest

As a concept, legitimating inactivity similarly demonstrates these intensified self-policing and self-regulatory practices in the management of the digital health self. More specifically, the users' perspectives resonated with Crawford's (1980s) theory of 'healthism', whereby 'health' becomes the prioritised aspect over all other focuses of life(style) for the individual subject. This was prevalent even in the cases when poor physical health prevented them from prioritising exercise. They felt frustrated and inadequate because of their inability to put 'healthy' behaviours into practice. This was especially evident in Sophie's case. Even though she had achieved her goal of running a marathon, she stated:

> 'I was gutted [I couldn't do more running] but then the only comfort I had from it was that I had just done the marathon so I felt like I had a good excuse, because everyone would be like "oh how's your running going?" so I was like "I've run the London marathon and my knee's bad."' (Sophie, final interview, 31, F)

> 'Spoke to a friend about my current (lack of) exercise regime. I'm frustrated as I can't do a lot at the moment. I'm always competitive with my peers. I need to minimise my sugar, and carb consumption to compensate for lack of movement.' (Matt, final interview, 41, M)

When usual exercise routines are not possible, different behaviours and exercises are adopted to maintain calorie burning, weight loss or personal development. Upon this adjustment, self-trackers often reflect the input versus output discourse we discussed in the earlier chapters and treat their body like a machine, which led to corresponding feelings of guilt for not reaching or working towards optimum fitness levels. Practices that are incomparable to previous behaviours are not identified as sufficient for progressing or even maintaining fitness levels. Rather, feelings of nostalgia towards previous 'levels' of fitness become the focal point of frustration at not being able to enact self-discipline and to 'improve'.

Managing and mediating between long-term and short-term 'health' goals is a key way to legitimate not undertaking acts that may prevent recovery. Users spoke of 'doing whatever you like' to keep up fitness, which does not refer to indulgence in 'treat' foods or inactivity. Rather, they spoke about wishing they could keep up exercise regimes to enable physical recovery from injury. Self-discipline, therefore, in this context shifts from the regulation of activity to the regulation of rest. This regulation seeks to ensure that if activity levels are lowered, this has to be internally 'legitimated' by self-trackers to achieve longer term or bigger goals. Achieving these bigger health goals (such as doing a marathon or achieving a yoga pose) authorised self-trackers to lower everyday fitness expenditure, to take time over what felt good for their body, rather than pushing through injury or discomfort due to their commitment or goal. For example, Lou enjoyed her yoga class in a different way after completing the marathon:

> 'Actually, now it's quite nice to take a step back and go to yoga and not be there because I should be stretching but because I want to go to yoga, going to different classes because I don't need to use that two-hour slot free going for a run.' (Lou, final interview, 29, F)

In this sense, on completion of her training regime and the London Marathon, she was able to enjoy other exercises for 'exercise's sake', without a goal to improve. This again demonstrates the proliferation of self-optimising and self-improvement discourses, which surround the use of self-tracking regulatory practices. Therefore, for many self-trackers the self becomes identifiable and related to through the self-management of its being (Foucault, 1988) and active responsible behaviours; inactivity, then, can often only be 'legitimated' through certain physical (in)capabilities.

Self-surveillance, shame and body image

Self-surveillance and the associated self-regulatory and disciplinary practices intensified when self-trackers became concerned over their body image being scrutinised by others. Body image is understood as the perception that a person has of their physical self and the thoughts and feelings that result from that perception (Shilder, 1935). These feelings can be positive, negative or both and are influenced by individual as well as environmental factors (Shilder, 1935). Whilst the study of technology's impact of body image is an interesting and evolving field, affective neuroscience literature, for example, has attended to this debate (see Panksepp, 2005; Tiggerman, 2011; Perloff, 2014). This book, however, is concerned with how self-surveillance and the associated tools that enable it, such as social media and self-tracking devices, affect users' perceptions through offline interactions with others, including peers, colleagues and even strangers:

> 'There was a couple of times after the gym where I've been into the co-op [supermarket] and I've picked up a ready meal because I couldn't be bothered to cook and then I bumped into someone from the gym and I actually just felt so guilty, and I was so embarrassed about what was in my basket.' (Sophie, final interview, 31, F)

For Sophie, this embarrassment about individual food choices and being 'caught' in the act of eating a 'cheat meal', for example, ties into discourses of shame around a lack of commitment to certain 'health' practices, a mismanagement of health or a lack of self-discipline. These findings reflect Kristensen et al's (2016) research, which examined how food choices and in particular shopping baskets offered insights into the moral character of citizens and how this may be perceived, presented or performed, illustrating

Cederstrom and Spicer's (2015: 7) argument that 'eating has become a paranoid activity (…) It puts your identity to the test.' This is also intensified by talking extensively about goals or challenges to friends, family or colleagues, as well as by posting regularly about your diet, which ensures there is a front to maintain: a façade of a 'healthy self'. In this way, Sophie also felt a huge pressure from her gym community and social circle to look a 'certain way'. As argued by Heyes (2006: 126), 'people diet because they act on false beliefs about the possibility and desirability of losing weight for the sake of their health', physical appearance and performing physical transformations. Sophie spoke openly about a 12-week challenge, which involved dieting and specific exercises, and was concerned that those she had spoken to would expect her to look 'transformed':

> I wish I hadn't told anyone I was doing this challenge because I feel like I've put too much pressure on myself to look good enough at the end of it and also what food I am seen to be eating. If no one knew about it then they wouldn't be looking at me and expecting me to look a certain way. (Sophie, diary entry, 31, F)

Being a healthy role model was an identity that many self-trackers embodied. Whilst they gained positive feelings from this recognition from their peers, it also contrasted with feelings of internalised pressure to behave and perform in certain ways. Foucault (1984: 27) understands this as 'assujettissement': the process of at once becoming a subject and becoming subjected. This is emphasised through these technologies, whereby health and identity management amongst online and offline networks becomes an ongoing consideration for self-trackers who regularly shared their lives on social media. In turn, lifestyle becomes representative of body image, while self-identification is achieved through self-transformation and life-strategising technologies, which enable one to compete within a community, and is further encouraged through self-tracking practices (Urry and Elliot, 2010).

> I feel I have a reputation amongst friends for being fit, healthy and strong and therefore feel responsible for sharing my lifestyle in an attempt to inspire, motivate and lift others up with me. Which in turn helps me with my internal goals of health and fitness. (Annie, diary entry, 28, F)

Self-trackers who regularly performed their healthy self frequently spoke about a pressure to look 'good enough' or a 'certain way', which was usually in comparison to how their peers around them would perceive their body image. This ideology often operated through oppressive patriarchal discourses of fat shaming, myths around what constitutes 'good' health and weight, and idealised and objectified body shapes (Heyes, 2006). For female users, wanting to look a 'certain way' also sat in line with the aesthetic heteronormative visual representations of the female body on Instagram: a slender, fit, gaze of a sexualised and idealised body shape (Elias and Gill, 2016). Interestingly, very few male participants raised concerns about their body image or how they were physically perceived, both online and offline. The male self-trackers tended to become concerned about weight gain and body image when they were unable to exercise due to illness. However, all the female users spoke about concern over how their body was perceived, supporting a wealth of literature that identifies the negative impact of Instagram on (female) body image (Facebook, 2021). For example, one of the users, Lara, frequently spoke about how she compared herself to other Chamonix residents: 'Chamonix is full of a lot of healthy athletes and hearing their stories is inspiring, I always feel well below par compared to them' (Lara, diary entry, 28, F).

In her final interview, Lara explained how she would not feel as much pressure to be so active if she were living in a large city (London, for example) that was not focused on seasonal sports such as skiing, snowboarding and mountain biking, as Chamonix is. Physical location, as well as seeing others' 'active' lives online, leads self-trackers to compare themselves and their fitness levels to others in their geographic location:

> 'A friend and I found out another group of girls have been rude about us and our "outdoorsy- ness" or lack of it in their eyes, and how much we drink. I've always kept myself surrounded by people who are mostly uplifting of each other so was a bit annoyed by these comments (…) I do feel it has an impact on how you view yourself and your health. I think I'm quite comfortable in my own skin. Obviously, there are things I'd like to improve upon, but that comes from myself, not from others' views. Having said that, I do feel an element of pressure to prove them wrong.' (Lara, final interview, 29, F)

This extract demonstrates how much others' poor perception of one's body image can dramatically impact on that individual's self-esteem, sense of self-worth and personal health identity. Prior to hearing about these derogatory comments from other peers and 'friends' in Chamonix, Lara felt confident about her body and 'health'. She acknowledges that there are aspects she would like to 'improve' but the desire to do so comes from (to an extent) her own goals, rather than pressure or comments from others. Once she hears (by word of mouth) that other women perceive her and her social circle to be 'unhealthy' (heavy drinkers of alcohol) and inactive, she feels a desire to want to change their perception of her as it does not line up with or mirror how she perceives herself. This continuous reflexive and self-evaluative cycle also incorporates a simultaneous consideration of upholding or amending others' potential judgements of their personal body image by incorporating more regulatory or disciplinary practices in management of their digital health self. This highlights the neoliberal shift towards obsessions and moral judgement and scorn of others' sliding morals (LeBesco, 2011: 72). In response to potential or actual moral scorn, self-trackers were continually self-evaluative, which led to a constant self-surveillance, as well as regulation and discipline related to consumption, exercise and any health-related practices. Lifestyle change or 'lifestyle correction' (Leichter, 1997: 359) is often considered the only way to respond to perceived poor body image. The practices adopted and the self-presentation moulded or constructed in consideration of imagined judgements from the wider social media and offline community are examined in more detail in Chapters 3 and 6.

Disciplining the 'healthy role model'

Enacting healthy living for the benefit of others was a challenge that self-trackers related to being a 'role model', whilst simultaneously attempting not to instil their self-policing pressures on others. This 'aim' to present oneself by way of being an 'example' to others could be conceived as a way of legitimating narcissistic practices of self-representation. Yet users who placed a huge amount of self-regulation upon themselves (and corresponding feelings of shame or guilt if not maintained) did feel a desire to prevent their networks (online and offline) from embodying those same pressures. As Sophie stated:

> It's really shallow but I'm going [to Ibiza] with a group of girls and if I'm honest they look up to me, they look at me as the fitness, healthy one, I hate it when they come to ask me is this ok to eat. (Sophie, diary entry, 31, F)

> 'It's so much pressure. It's like, we're going with Sophie one of my friends was like "you're so skinny", I don't want to be skinny.' (Sophie, final interview, 31, F)

Interestingly, the participants became experts in identifying and reflecting upon their own self-policing practices, whilst trying to protect and shield those in their social circle who admired their behaviours from adopting the same negative self-policing and self-regulation, which arguably damaged their self-esteem. These reflexive and disciplinary practices lead to the creation of a self-surveying subject, who attempts to 'discipline' an 'unruly' body (Gill, 2007a: 152) and then represents that transformative struggle for the benefit of guiding others. This places pressures on self-trackers to be seen as 'the healthy one' by their friends and colleagues. In addition to being seen as health or fitness 'obsessed', the stigmas attached to being skinny are a concern for users. Being skinny is often associated with eating disorders, and therefore poor mental and physical health, which these participants categorically do not want to be associated with. Sophie has suffered with bulimia in the past and spoke about feeling like a 'fake':

> 'I had an eating disorder, I was binging because I was feeling depressed (…) then I was like I shouldn't have eaten this, then I was making myself sick and throwing it up. I can talk about it, it's fine, but I was like "oh I'm a massive fake."' (Sophie, final interview, 31, F)

Being slim and controlling calories were assumed to demonstrate 'acts of health' (Goodyear et al, 2017: 7), reflecting an oversimplification of the representation of a 'healthy body – the lean, toned body – as a signifier of moral worth. (…) a necessary step towards health' (LeBesco 2011: 81). Sophie felt comfortable discussing her eating disorder with the researcher, in the private interview space. Since she had a serious health disorder she felt like a 'fraud' to her friends, family and colleagues, as she was promoting her 'healthy' lifestyle to them whilst still struggling with this disease. Sophie did not consider herself to be 'in recovery' from this illness, but she still embodied feelings of regret and remorse, as well as anxiety about her perceived lack of self-discipline since she could not 'overcome' this illness. In this way, representing herself as the 'healthy one' to friends, family and colleagues could be conceived as an arguable way for her to emotionally compensate for her guilt associated with her illness.

Burdens of disciplinary self-tracking

This section analyses in depth the burden of disciplinary self-tracking related to the intensified practices of self-policing, regulation and the moralism of 'health', which users increasingly embodied over time. The existing literature on this topic associates disadvantage with personal failure (Sayar, 2004; Cederstrom and Spicer, 2015). However, I argue that using these devices and platforms further entrenches personal failure within discourses of poor self-discipline and poor 'health' self-management, particularly in the context of neoliberalism's power over self-perception of the body (Brandt and Rozin, 1997). To put it in new materialistic terms, the mind controls individual behaviours, and responsibilities are internally practiced and maintained (Moore and Robinson, 2016). This can be exemplified in the research findings when users felt the practices of self-tracking were becoming tiresome and burdensome:

> I guess I felt that my daily commute is stressful enough to add another thing to it. I know it was only a weekly progress, but on Mondays

> I knew I was going to share after my commute, I just had enough and no longer wanted to be burdened by it. (Fet, diary entry, 30, M)

This user shared his commute only once a week to self-survey, track and share progress with his social media community. A few months after relocating, the struggles related to commuting, as well as self-tracking, felt like a burden that had outweighed its previously interpreted 'benefits' of capturing, for example, elevation, time and speed. Self-trackers also felt frustrated when they could neither undertake their fitness practices nor acquire the relevant data:

> I felt a little dissatisfied at myself for getting up slightly late today and being unable to post (...) I knew the following week will be a week off work and I would have liked to gain some sort of data of my time prior to a week off, especially as I had a week off previously due to wet weather. (Fet, diary entry, 30, M)

From this extract we see how discourses of data acquisition become tied to self-worth and attribute personal satisfaction to acquiring data-driven constructions of the self. In this practice sensor quantification and data acquisition become representative of 'health' – more than human instincts – which do not take into consideration senses that cannot be measured (feelings or instincts). In essence, it does not consider the elements that set us apart from computers, as human beings. For example, Fet did not express frustration at not being able to cycle to work as he overslept but was rather disappointed that he could not acquire the data from his commute. Since he would be on annual leave the following week, and the previous week he could not cycle due to bad weather, he desired to acquire data to ensure that there were no 'gaps' is his data capture and representation on his 'Map My Ride' application. Purpura et al (2011: 6) consider there to be 'issues around surveillance and the ascendancy of data collection over personal experience as a means for establishing truth and manipulating behaviour'. In this regard, Fet felt frustrated at not being able to track his cycle ride. Although he completed his commute, he craved the data to represent it. Therefore, self-tracking and quantification reduce human 'health' to numbers and patterns, through code mediated by algorithms, and often it is that reductive data representation of 'health' that self-trackers desire to seek over health improvements. Therefore, statistics can become a priority over human instinct and personal health decisions. The self-tracking device or social media platform can only represent what it does know and not what it does not. In this regard, this monograph extensively argues that it is imperative for application, device and platform developers and consumers to realise that good health cannot be simply attributed to data (Taleb, 2012).

Knowing how many calories you consumed, or whether you slept badly or ran slowly, does not provide the self-tracker with anything more than that information. This oversimplification without context dehumanises the user and turns them into to a 'good' or 'bad' number, which is restrictive in that you cannot provide context related to external lifestyle factors. This became particularly problematic when taking into consideration disease and mental health issues, especially for those who struggled with their relationship with food and those with eating disorders. Sophie's diary entry was contextualised further in her final interview:

> 'So, I've made a conscious decision to write on this day when I haven't posted any pictures, more specifically food pictures as I feel like I need a break from posting as much food stuff.' (Sophie, final interview, 31, F)

Deciding to take a break from self-tracking and sharing health content made users feel protected; posting over time turns their gaze further inward, intensifying practices of self-discipline and regulation. Users identified this self-policing as damaging to their mental health. Upon reflection, when interrogating this process personally, these users felt that self-tracking either quantitatively, through biometric data capture applications, or qualitatively, through 'selfies' or food photography, felt regulatory and provided forbidding (though self-proclaimed) boundaries. This perspective resonated with Purpura et al's (2011: 6) assertion that 'while personal goals are always culturally influenced, the key distinguishing feature (…) is that users do not get to choose their own viewpoints but are provided with one by designers'. The ability of humans to intervene when it comes to the damaging effects of such devices and platforms is limited as one can monitor or quantify only within the limitations or challenges decided by the application. This is achieved by 'pulling quantitative measures to the foreground over qualitative ones and usurping the normal situational human decision-making process' (Purpura et al, 2011: 7). A sense of 'empowerment' and being 'free' was a common discourse associated with not using these devices and not self-tracking:

> 'My phone [battery] died when I was running. I took out my headphones and I could hear the birds and the trees rustling and it was actually quite nice. I always thought I needed the music to keep me going and giving me a bit of a boost, but I was ok actually. I did the 10 km without my phone. You don't know what time you're doing. You don't know how fast you're running. You're just doing what you can. Before, I found the Nike app really annoying, I found it a bit slow because each time I kind of knew when I was going to be getting to the 1 or 2-mile mark and it was like it doesn't know where

> it is, because it's slow and it kept changing it. It was also like telling me the time and the next time, and I'd been working out in my head like "you're going slower now". It couldn't figure out how I'd been slower or faster, and I can't feel like I can go any faster because I'm doing what I can but I'm now feeling the pressure from the app to do better (…) My phone's not get much memory so I just deleted it in the end.' (Lara, final interview, 28, F)

Users were irritated by technical issues, the fallibility of the apps and the short battery life or memory of a smartphone or self-tracking device. However, this was at times interpreted as a positive by-product of using these devices, releasing the participant from the shackles of self-tracking and self-discipline. As Lara described, the joy of not monitoring enabled her to appreciate nature, hearing the birds and the trees rustling around her. Not relying on something to track her movement enabled her to be present in the moment without the distraction and accompaniment of a phone or device. Lara reflected that she felt she would need music on her phone and the tracking device to motivate her to keep going, but interestingly without it she simply enjoyed the process of running without external influences. Therefore, persuasive computing and the data that is produced by self-tracking applications have various functions, which could be considered coercion rather than encouragement. As Giroux (2014: xvi) asserts:

> As a mode of governance, it produces identities, subjects, and ways of life driven by a survival-of-the fittest ethic, grounded in the idea of the free, possessive individual, and committed to the right of ruling groups and institutions to exercise power removed from matters of ethics and social costs.

Using the tracking device pressured Lara to 'do better', 'be fitter' and keep going against all costs, which felt over-regulatory, so much so that she deleted the app. Notably, she recognised that without her phone and tracking app 'you're just doing what you can', demonstrating the proliferation of self-optimisation discourses surrounding these technologies, devices and platforms, as well as the pressure to share these quantified captures of exercise, 'health' practices and personal experience. This begs the question: Do we do much anymore without considering its captured and represented counterpart? For anyone who tracks or life-logs in this way, this query extends further than health or fitness-related content and becomes centred around the continual self-representation of life(style), personal activities and behaviours. As Lupton (2013e: 11) recognises, the 'mundane aspects of one's life are constantly shared with others, including those that may previously have been kept private'. Although users self-surveyed through self-tracking, as well as their physical movements and consumption practices (food and drink intake), their motivations for doing so were at times lost within regimented self-regulatory processes:

> 'The training plan becomes a bit of a weird thing. I obviously wanted to run the marathon and I entered it for myself but then actually you've got this plan to follow so it becomes a bit regimented.' (Lou, final interview, 29, F)

Lou was using 'Map My Run' to track her marathon training plan and realised over many months of using this application that she actually found it quite restrictive and self-regulatory. At times it felt overwhelming and distracted her from her personal goal of marathon training. This reflects a common discourse that features throughout the research findings, in which the process of self-surveillance through self-tracking personal activity sometimes removed the goal of what users were hoping to individually achieve, and thus the acquisition of data frequently becomes the new goal. This perspective resonates with Lupton's (2012b: 237) argument that 'the body is hardly able to disappear when its functions, movements, and habits are constantly monitored, and the user of m-health technologies is made continually aware, via feedback, of these dispositions'. This continual feedback from data acquired by self-trackers was identified as motivating for training; however, they also felt it was over-policing, in a negative regulatory way. The app reminding the users of the time left to run was far from encouraging but was rather demotivating. Therefore, the application can be seen as capable of limiting or extending human capabilities depending upon the goals provided by the device. This form of persuasive computing encourages a scientific rationalisation of our everyday lives. Regardless of personal circumstances or external factors, it 'values quantification and rationality at the cost of situational, hard-to-measure factors and sees scientific measurement as obviating personal experience' (Purpura et al, 2011: 6). This discourse argues that self-quantification reduces human activity and behaviours to numbers, to a human version of computing that does not take into consideration all human senses and attributes. Being continually notified and 'nudged' by the app of the time and distance left to go can remind the user of the challenges ahead, which may not be achieved, and can cause anxiety. Furthermore, the optimisation of the self-improvement cycle never ends and holds as much weight (in terms of acknowledging personal fitness development) for the individual as the actual physical improvement:

> 'There was a time when I would've looked at me now and been well happy with it but now I think I look at a lot of pictures of people online

> and even though I know they're photo-shopped I feel like I need to look like that, I need abs like that, I need my arms to look like that.' (Sophie, final interview, 31, F)

We see in this extract that self-optimisation goals and practices rarely culminate. Self-trackers express a commitment to the continuing nature of self-tracking, monitoring and community surveillance cultures, where goals and comparisons may never be reached. This could damage self-esteem through feelings of failure or inadequacy when comparing themselves to others. As Thacker (2003: 56) describes in his theory of cultural attitudes towards the body and bio-media more broadly: 'our culture wants to render the body immediate, while also multiplying our capacity to technically control the body.' The immediacy of the body is enabled for Lou in the earlier quote, through the regulatory design 'nudges' reminding her of the distance to go. App developers would argue that these socio-technological affordances motivate the user. However, as demonstrated here, this sometimes fails, as this 'nudge' is interpreted as controlling and at times demotivating. This challenges dominant discourses around these consumer products, which stipulate that self-tracking devices support and enable 'healthier' decisions and 'healthier' bodies. However, in practice, the body is not a machine and cannot be technologically 'controlled', managed or 'optimised' in this way, and anxieties, guilt and shame arise when the moralisation of health is internalised in this way.

Conclusions

As this chapter has shown, self-tracking is not just about the technology but rather about what it means when people use these technologies and the physical, mental or emotional changes that occur (Butterfield, 2012). Over time, morality, 'health' and body image often become inextricably linked to practices of disciplinary self-tracking, associated with accumulated data and subsequent data constructions of the self (see Figure 4.1). Self-tracking devices may provide individuals with 'information' about their bodies, but such quantification cannot extend to the human mind, instincts and intuition or take into consideration external factors that cannot be quantified. These computer sensors cannot factor in the unquantifiable. When one is unwell, for example, should the user respond to their application when a 'run reminder' alerts them on their device? These 'unintended' consequences or eventualities can lead to controlling behaviours through coding and algorithms, removing the inherently important role of human senses and prioritising technological sensors. Of course, the human body and mind cannot be reduced solely in this way, and quantifying and tracking one's life can only provide the user with limited

Figure 4.1: Example of participant-shared self-tracking content

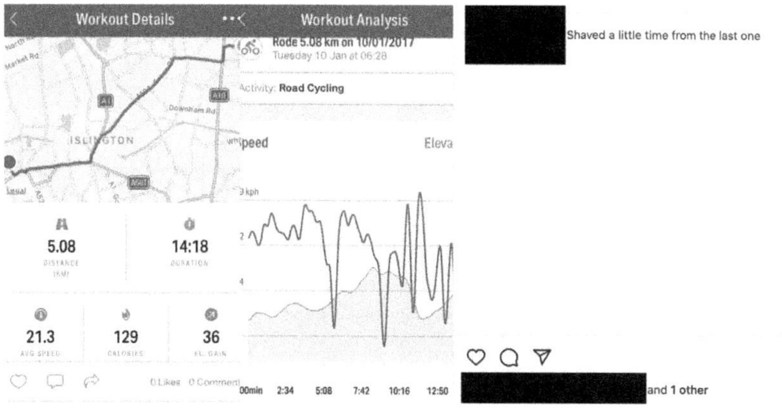

'information'. What therefore becomes important within these dictating technological frames is the need to re-learn and remind ourselves to trust human instinct, as well as to ask ourselves how healthy, unwell or tired we feel. As Leriche and Arnulf famously wrote in 1936 (73, 6.16–1), 'health is [often] lived in the silence of the organs.' Disease and ill health therefore embody states of suffering, and it is the individuals who distinguish this state (disease) from normal health, viewing it as pathological, as it is they who are suffering from it.

Individuals adhere to citizenship responsibilities of good 'health' and good morality so as not to be a 'burden' to the state and society, as well as to identify as 'belonging' citizens. These findings argue that good health cannot be simply attributed to data. As Taleb (2012: np) understands it: 'asking science to explain life and vital matters is equivalent to asking a grammarian to explain poetry.' There are limitations on any level of expertise, especially one that relies upon technological sensors, number quantification or representation, which cannot take into consideration many external and human factors. Self-tracking devices, apps and social media platforms can be positioned and understood by users as a technology of the self, further enabling and expanding health management capacities (Rose, 1999; Ajana, 2005), which problematically links personal lifestyle choices and health decisions to consumer-led solutions. Not everything in our body can be systematised or managed through datafication. The mind, body, health and the soul of an individual cannot be wholly reduced to data. We might then return to LeBesco's (2011) arguments and avoid using phrases such as 'healthy weight', as they bestow moral as well as aesthetic value on slim bodies. In reality, a wide variety of body shapes and sizes could be 'healthy weights' for those individuals, the point being that it is not possible to illustrate or exemplify good health just by looking at someone or their data.

Therefore, it must be recognised that these practices are limited in the extent to which they can enable or promote good 'health'. This problematic convergence of the body and technology through health, fitness and lifestyle tracking is an inherent self-governing and self-regulatory practice, which deeply permeated the everyday lives of the participants, even if (in)action did not correspond to associated interpretations of pride, elation, anxiety, immorality, guilt or shame. From this it can be said that the participants' personal decision-making and thought processes, feelings and embodiments are self-governing, self-evaluative and thus deeply self-disciplined. Even when technology is removed entirely or resisted in these self-disciplinary self-tracking cultures, the regulation of the body, with or without the tools and technologies of the self, is still prevalent, preventative and self-policing in the mind of the user (Moore and Robinson, 2016). Whilst this chapter has explored many different aspects, practices and considerations related to self-tracking and discipline and moralism, it is clear that the overarching dominant discourse, ideology and all-encompassing theme throughout are that of regulation: of the self and identity, technology, the body and the mind, and the convergence of all these aspects through various self-tracking technological devices, wearables, applications and platforms. Therefore, using self-tracking technology and social media as health management tools has made individual ethics become somatic, leading to a pervasive moralism of everyday 'health'.

5

Health 'Disciples': Technology 'Addiction' and Embodiment

This chapter explores shifting social media and self-tracking sharing and performative etiquettes over time, including practices of both technological compulsions and 'addiction' (Dong and Potenza, 2014; Alter, 2107; He et al, 2017), as well as the complexities around narratives and practices of digital detoxing (Kent, 2020a). Through analysis of the empirical data (interviews, reflexive diaries and online content), this chapter examines how and why users digitally detox from self-tracking (devices) and social media platforms for a time or indeed quit them altogether. This chapter presents users' perceived burdens of self-tracking and the self-regulation promoted by these technologies: how they can become emotionally detrimental to users' sense of wellbeing, mental and physical health. It is through the ubiquity of mediated identity that individuals represent and mould their diets and bodies to the desired aesthetics on social media (Kent, 2020b) and become self-proclaimed disciples of 'health' (Kent, 2018). This chapter looks at these practices in detail, from users becoming 'lay experts' of health in their striving for health knowledge, to the technical issues they can face during this self-policing knowledge cycle, to related compulsive practices and 'addictive' behaviours, to burdens of being a health disciple and practices of digital detox. We begin with a detailed definition of a health disciple.

Health 'disciples'

> 'I was like a disciple, and I still am (…) It's in my psyche now (…) I went through two months where I did no exercise, but it kept me in that kind of mind-set. (…) There was always a slight influence of health.' (Jennie, first interview, 40, F)

Being a 'disciple' of health means capturing and sharing health-related content simultaneously, which over time becomes both a conscious and an unconscious desire. The focus on 'healthiness' dominates these users' everyday lives; even if they are not able to maintain 'healthy' behaviours, health disciples genuinely identified with being a healthy person due to past self-tracking and representational behaviours. Regardless of their current behaviours, the 'health self' was continually embodied by self-trackers (Kent, 2018: 62). The 'health self is an all-encompassing healthy identity which permeated their sense of being in the world. Users often automatically shared self-tracked 'personal bests' on social media. Achieving certain goals (for example, time or distances), either individually or competitively within the online community, was considered 'good enough' to be shared because it demonstrated such individual improvement. These types of data sharing resonate with van Dijck's (2014) theories of 'dataism', which refers to a pervasive belief in objective quantification, tracking and logging of all kinds of human behaviour and sociality through technology. For example, Sophie stated, whilst marathon training,

> 'Because of sharing, you've got to get a certain time and obviously, you want to get a good time in the marathon, but you'd be stopping at a road because there's traffic. You'd be stressing out because it's going to affect your time. So, you'd be thinking you've got to run this last bit faster because of the time (…) You still knew you run well, you know that on the day there won't be traffic. But you just get obsessed with posting it.' (Sophie, first interview, 31, F)

Whilst training for exercise goals is important, what becomes increasingly prioritised for many self-trackers is the capturing of the goal time or distance on the application and adjusting exercise to meet this. Not only did tracking and improving upon time and distance become a key demonstration of self-maintenance through individual regulation and self-improvement, but genuine frustrations of the 'real' or offline world (stopping at a pedestrian crossing) affected overall statistics of goals set by users and produced emotionally embodied pressures. Additionally, fallibility of the apps, when data was lost or incorrectly captured, is a real concern for self-trackers. The representation of data can carry weight and significance over users' sense of personal gratification. At times, however, faulty devices or inaccurate data can work in favour of these 'idealised' representations. For instance, if a faulty device captures what is determined by the user as an improved time or speed, this is considered as a positive representation, however inaccurate and false that representation may be. In line with 'dataism' (van Dijck, 2014), these practices reflect Ruckenstein's (2014) research on the significance of data visualisations, interpreted by users as more 'factual', or 'credible', insights into their daily lives than their subjective experiences. This similarly reflected the cultural notion that 'seeing' makes knowledge reliable and trustworthy

(Ruckenstein, 2014) and often reinforced their 'winning and achieving at all costs' mentality (Goodyear et al, 2017: 8). We can see these practices as a consistent commitment to 'healthism' (Crawford, 1980) mediated by their relationships to technology; this ensured that health priorities fed into many other areas of lifestyle, which contributed to feelings of personal achievement, self-worth and happiness.

What can be extended from 'healthism' (Crawford, 1980) in these practices is the striving towards and the embodiment of becoming a disciple. Accumulated tracked or shared data and health-related content become the users' 'digital health self'; both ideologically and due to self-representations online, the accrual of both shared qualitative and quantitative health content ensures a user conceives of their commitment to healthism (and arguably 'dataism') regardless of current behaviours. For example, even if healthy practices have stopped, the 'disciple' ideology and mentality of users still exist firmly in the minds of those who strive towards a digital health self both mentally and physically, regardless of what they are consuming or a lack of exercise. The past tracked data and representation of a user's 'digital health self' and celebrated achievements via perceptions of 'objective' truth telling data illustrate self-improvement, and once accumulated over time, this is the core mentality of the 'disciple' of the health self. It is also worth recognising this desire for self-optimisation within a neoliberal framework of choice architecture and self-motivation, this arguable individual health virtue becomes signalled via the performance online of being a disciple of health. As Lupton (2006: 240) highlights:

> Individuals make choices not in a social vacuum, but in a context in which certain kinds of subjects and bodies are privileged over others (...) the responsible, self-disciplined body/self (...) who is interested in and motivated to improve their health.

For these 'health disciples', identifying as 'healthy' is the mantra for and is often prioritised over most if not all aspects of life(style) (Cederstrom and Spicer, 2015). The produced 'data double', which refers to the reductionist representation of the monitored body as data (Whitson and Haggerty, 2008: 574; Moore, 2017), could be conceived as providing the participants with more than a one-dimensional visual engagement with their bodies. Rather than simply visualising their previously tracked activities, exercises or 'healthy behaviours', which could lead to feelings of guilt if current behaviours were not reflective of this, this self-tracked representation on their devices provided participants with a 'datafication of health' that they still embodied and related to and because of which they felt 'healthy'. In addition, being a health 'disciple' also meant prioritising research on your chosen health discipline (fitness or food oriented) to develop a level of expertise. This process can be understood as becoming a 'lay expert' of health.

'Lay expertise' of health and its history

Firstly, we shall draw upon medical sociology literature for this book's definition and application of the term 'lay expertise'. We outlined in Chapter 1, 'Transformations of Health in the Digital Society', how doctors and medical staff in the National Health Service were seen as 'medical prestige' and health expertise in the eyes of the public (Seale, 2003). This relationship was extremely paternalistic, in that clinical expertise was conceived of as a powerful role, unquestioned by passive and 'unknowing' patients (Anderson and Gillam, 2001). Bensaude-Vincent (2016: 1) argued that the 'radical disqualification of the public goes hand in hand with claims of a radical break between quantum physics or relativity theory and common sense. The more recent movements of citizen science and participatory science testify to a radical change in the relation between expert knowledge and lay knowledge.' The practice of 'lay expertise' in the assessment of scientific credibility has a history identifiable back to the fitness and nutritional science boom of the 1970s and 1980s, whereby links between diet and health became widely understood by the general public. The development of clinical research and nutritional science during this time (Mennel, 1992; Brandt and Rozin, 1997) was also associated with an increase in British press coverage of 'health issues' (Williams and Miller, 1998). We can conceive of this shift, from the dynamic of paternalism between clinicians and patients to patients seeking out their own health guidance, as one of the first developments of lay expertise in health self-management on a broad societal level. A heightened awareness of the science of 'health' developed, which reconsidered the socio-economic impact upon health rather than just focusing on 'bad' food consumption in the development of ill health. This increase in knowledge about nutritional and health sciences has encouraged the development of the self-help movement, and political priorities shifted towards the needs of the individual rather than the rights of the whole society (Anderson and Gillam, 2001).

Arguably, we can conceive of self-help as the initial motivator (due to wider neoliberal socio-cultural and economic shifts) that promoted self-knowledge for health management. Lay expertise then, is about seeking credibility, which combines aspects of power, dependence, legitimation, persuasion and trust (Weber, 1978) and which is about not just social authority but also cultural authority resting upon an individual's capacity to offer what is considered to be a 'truth' (Starr, 1982: 13). Credibility, therefore, is the backbone of the moral order in modern scientific inquiry and trust (Shapin, 1994). Therefore, lay expertise can occur where there is a credibility gap or if solutions do not yet exist or are not yet presented (Epstein, 2004). This was clearly witnessed during the early months of COVID-19 (Kent, 2021) as the public waded through a wealth of health, wellness and COVID-19 guidance and tips on social media, 'turning most of us into medical lay experts continually attempting to decipher between what is legitimate information and what is nonsense' (Kent, 2021: np.). This is further explored in Chapter 7, 'Future Directions for the Digital Health Self'. Over the course of this chapter, we examine examples that illustrate this rise of the lay expert, broadly due to several socio-cultural, economic and political factors and, in particular, the shift towards neoliberalism and healthism.

Developing lay expertise for the digital health self

When frequent users of self-tracking tools share a data representation (both qualitative and quantitative) of their 'health' and lifestyle on social media, they battled with the hybridity of what they understood as personal, private and self-representational online identities. At what point, under the gaze of the online community, did they become experienced in their health identity as a yogi, a runner or a cyclist, for example? What now qualifies as a health or exercise expert in data-sharing cultures – especially when considering that many of these users are not medically trained, qualified or sharing credible medical guidance or advice but representations of a healthy lifestyle? How can we determine what is 'healthy' information or misinformation? As has been outlined in earlier chapters, it has now been widely reported the challenges many of us face when attempting to identify reliable health information online, and social media is often relied upon for health guidance, over the NHS online resources for example (Plaisime et al, 2020). This is a huge problem, which regulators and legislators have been grappling with and will continue to grapple with for many years to come.

So how does this manifest for self-trackers? This becomes an especially pertinent question when those simply sharing their 'digital health self' online are not doing so for monetary gain, or to influence the behaviour of others, but simply to share their daily activities for motivation, support, accountability and appreciation. However, in time these non-intentional influencers may become a figure of influence within their social networks and, in turn, a role model for others. Even those with best intentions to not directly influence others' behaviours or consumption practices can in time become an influencer of sorts, even without commercially motivated sharing. Frequent sharers still often conform to the conventions and representational logics of influencer culture and commodification of the self. These trends and practices are further analysed in Chapter 6, but for now, let us analyse the tensions of online identity for frequent, and arguably compulsive, health content sharers. It can be asked then: What does it mean to cycle for pleasure as well as practical purposes such as cycling to work? What does it mean to enjoy cycling without feeling a desire to document its benefits online, whilst at other times sharing self-tracked cycling data? What different identities are embodied when exercising as part of a commuting routine and exercising for fun, competitively or as a group activity? If scientific knowledge induces power relations (Bensaude-Vincent, 2016), and self-tracking of the body is a type (albeit problematic) of scientific data, then what does it mean to use that data for health improvement or to reach training goals? Where does the expertise and/or authority lie, for example, between being a (non-professional) marathon runner and being someone who runs for pleasure and to keep fit? These questions are pertinent when considering the narrative of many self-trackers and their sharing. One of the participants, Lou, was training for the London Marathon; as the event neared and her training advanced, her identity as a 'layperson' marathon trainer shifted into becoming a 'marathon runner': 'It felt like I really was a marathon runner (to be!)' (Lou, diary entry, 29, F).

The social media sharing of these activities and particularly developments is a key component to legitimating athlete-like or developments towards 'expert' health and fitness identities. Lou's perceptions shifted from being someone who ran for pleasure and to keep fit to someone who was running for a definitive purpose due to her commitment to the running event, as well as her accumulated running representation and development documented on social media. In this regard, this participant's self-perception of increasing her 'expertise' to not only take part but compete in the marathon. A level of expertise, then, is gained through Lou's perceptions of her own health identity, which transformed into a more 'professional' conceptualisation of self and health activity that considered the 'impressive' increasing capabilities of her body. This illustrates a credibility shift from someone whose goal is to run a marathon to entering a credibility arena of marathon runners via self-tracking her training. Entering this 'credibility arena' via tracked data legitimates the users' expertise, which in this field arguably transforms the very definition of what counts as credibility (Bensaude-Vincent, 2016: 409).

'Credibility arena' of health/fitness (micro-)influencers

Users regularly view other social media sharers (we could see them as 'micro-influencers', perhaps) as motivating figures who provide inspirational content but sometimes felt intimidated by their achievements. Feelings of intimidation usually had a demotivating impact. Other users felt that 'professional' or 'expert' levels of achievement or knowledge were unattainable, even though the 'influencers' they followed were rarely professional athletes or qualified dietitians, just individuals who presented and commodified themselves as such to legitimate and brand their 'coaching' and knowledge sharing to gain followers. In fact, research by the University of Glasgow recently found that 90 per cent of weight management advice shared by 'influencers' is inaccurate (Sabbagh et al, 2020), and yet users frequently interpret this information as credible, legitimate and a goal to aspire towards. This is especially demonstrated by participants who identified as runners but who compared themselves to 'better' or professional runners as a motivating exercise tool:

> 'This time round I managed to go further in my training runs. I was quicker in my training runs, so I think I actually felt a bit more like, even though I wouldn't classify myself as a runner compared to a lot of my friends even though they think I am because I've run quite a lot, but I'm nowhere near professional or anything like that. But I definitely felt more prepared and ready for it this time. It was probably the sort of thing I would never get to mentally in my head if I wasn't reflecting on it and writing it down [in the reflexive diary]. I don't think there was any moment when I was like you're totally Mo Farah, you've totally got this.' (Lou, final interview, 29 F)

To unpack Lou's self-identification in Giddens' (1991) terms, it can be said that Lou supplies herself with a biography and a personal narrative that express her enjoyment of running regularly but not being a professional. Yet, through comparative dialogue and discussion with others, and the additional self-reflexivity displayed in the diarising, Lou draws on these narratives and identities and thus embodies being a fit, active and proficient runner capable of achieving her goals. Another participant, Matt, further draws on this comparison and the continual competition arguably inherent in fitness communities. He explains that for him the comparison affects his sense of identity and personal achievement, and argues:

> 'Whatever you do regardless of what you do there's always going to be someone that's fitter, faster or stronger than you, so basically the only person that you are actually in competition with is yourself.' (Matt, final interview, 41, M)

Sense of self was not individually interpreted by these users as what one is born with, but it was about (neoliberal) self-transformation (Leichter, 1997). Like Giddens' (1991) theories of the self, the participants I worked with had a sense of self that was not fixed and bounded; it changed over time. One's sense of self, therefore, was not considered to be something permanent but was conceptualised as a transformative entity, continually evolving, with self-transformation becoming a lifestyle approach for many self-trackers. Even if many users chose not to describe it in this way, most considered these practices and inherent self-reflexive evaluations as a 'way of life'. In this regard, the 'self' is a reflexive project, which is continually worked and reflected upon (Giddens, 1991). The self does not exist without being continually monitored, speculated upon and at times adjusted. In line with Giddens' (1991) arguments of identity being multifaceted yet whole, participants similarly saw their individual identity as complex but as one thing, which was part of a whole that needed to be improved upon:

> 'I do research it a lot, not necessarily on Instagram, but on the internet as a whole. I guess it's this sense of self that I still don't fully get. This is definitely something that I'll take away from this, it's something I want to know about and get to understand(…) I do kind of think of myself as being yogi if you will, but then I also don't, that's just something that I do (…) I do know who I am and am happy with who I am and all of that but I just couldn't really put that into words in that way.' (Tim, final interview, 34 M)

Arming oneself with a wealth of information satisfies anxieties for self-trackers that there may be blocks to understanding and self-improvement. The lay expert enters the arena of credibility in the mind of the self-tracker (Epstein, 2004), expressing a desire to research and learn more to strive to be the best version of themselves, reinforcing a discourse and cycle of continual learning and self-improvement. As Matt expressed, he frequently felt being in a 'mind-set of constantly trying to learn' (Matt, first interview, 41, M). This involved the '"strategic adoption of lifestyle options", likely to have been pulled from consumer culture, to relate to a planned "trajectory", geared to maintaining a meaningful biographical narrative' (Giddens, 1991: 243–244). The time spent on prioritising certain aspects of 'health' created an interesting dynamic for the self-trackers. There is much deliberation about what time should be allocated to doing which activity (exercise versus rest, or exercise versus preparing healthy food), demonstrating challenging health contentions for these individuals in their everyday lives. As Percey (1972: 113) asserts: 'In the lay culture of a scientific society, nothing is easier to fall prey to a kind of seduction which renders one's very self from itself into an all transcending "objective" consciousness and a consumer-self with a list of needs to be satisfied.' In recognition of not being of the same 'standard' as other health and fitness 'experts' online, many users spend a lot of their time researching their health and fitness interests to further their 'lay expertise'.

> 'It's almost to gain a bigger, wider understanding of it. So obviously I go to a yoga class, and I learn things and then that for me, for some people that would probably be enough and then they'd just go back

> next week and learn some more. For me I like to immerse myself in it and gain a bigger understanding for it, it probably enhances my sense of self I guess because without having a wide knowledge of it then I wouldn't feel that I was getting the most out of it as I could. For me that's important in lots of things that I do.' (Tim, final interview, 34, M)

Generating self-tracking data and sharing related content online further distance the data from lived experiences of users. Immaterial and disembodied characters of bio-media affect how we perceive the body and the biological realm (Thacker, 2003) and perhaps never more so than when we view other sharers' content of goals reached or bodily transformations on social media. Others' perceptions of individual parameters and the representation of disembodied characters can construct attainment in a distanced way, which, as the participants observed, may never be personally met:

> 'Initially I said I wanted to do a marathon and that's quite a big goal, so I think everyone was like "ummm". Then I thought " 'I'm going to try and prove you wrong" but obviously it was funny. One of the guys I work with, he wasn't encouraging, after doing the 10 km race was like yeah I think you're right, I should start with a half marathon, I don't want to go out into the full marathon.' (Lara, final interview, 28, F)

Other people's perceptions of their fitness levels, especially for beginners or people training towards a specific goal for the first time, feeds into users' own sense of what they felt they could achieve (or not). This sometimes manifested itself in quite a derogatory way, informed by negative feedback from their offline and online community when support for individual training was not received, as demonstrated in Lara's case. Therefore, these 'practices of surveillance, at the same time, entail and promote self-surveillance' (Goodyear et al, 2017: 3). As Rose (2007: 3) identifies, although 'grounded in norms and claims of truth (…) self-surveillance involves certain truths about how health and healthy behaviour is privileged'. These truth claims were often interpreted by the participants as having to be validated by external sources (Goodyear et al, 2017: 7). Confidence, then, is gained from commitment to goals, self-knowledge and expertise but also from satisfying all of one's personal choices, meaning good health becomes associated with individual choice (Leichter, 1997; Doshi, 2018). These lists do not centre around one goal but many, and self-achievement is felt and embodied only if all are satisfied. As Lara wrote:

> I felt really good and wanted to keep up the good routine of running regularly, doing more yoga and eating well. My mood was really good, I felt real sense of myself, like my confidence from the commitment

> I was making to myself was reassuring me somehow (…) I do find the more I make time for this for myself, the stronger I feel in myself to cope with other things. I find it really head clearing and affirmative in my own decision making. (Lara, diary entry, 28, F)

Self-tracking optimises this discourse of self-fulfilment being increasingly achievable through lay expertise, self-interested material and the ideological gain of the data, which is seen to provide legitimacy for their being and their role as a 'healthy' disciple of health and as a citizen, successfully self-regulating within a society of distanced state support; 'These aspects of diet and exercise can be seen as embodying broader cultural concerns (…) the emphasis of the attributes of efficiency, calculability, predictability, and nonhuman (frequently technological) control' (Purpura et al, 2011: 6–7). Users identified with a sense of control and self-discipline over the body, routines, health and fitness-related practices making them feel physically 'stronger' in themselves. This commitment to health expertise and self-management manifested itself as a personal responsibility and control over one's health, through the positive feelings associated with such actions, which over time become embodied and woven into the fabric of the digital health self.

Technological issues of being a 'health disciple'

As briefly covered in the previous section, diligently using self-tracking apps or devices provides users with fitness or health goals, but concerns are expressed when they feel regimented in some way. When the users were questioned during the interview to introspect these restrictions further, they identified the pressures they felt by using the applications were often resolved when they simply removed the tracking device from their health or fitness regimes. As demonstrated by Lara:

> I felt freer not using the app fully. Like I could just get on with it with no expectations, just take it for what it was. It was nice not having the music too for a change. (Lara, diary entry, 28, F)

Many users express feelings of being 'free' once they stopped using self-tracking devices, applications or social media. Contrastingly, when participants did want to use the technology to track 'health' and fitness-related activities, they were relieved when the device worked efficiently in tracking their movements. As Lou explained in her diary:

> Happy run was recorded. Relieved app hadn't crashed/ drained my phone battery on the run. Sense of completion. On training plan and for workout. (Lou, diary entry, 29, F)

> Satisfied I would be tracking our distance – to make sure we'd run far enough, but also a bit stressed that my phone would die part of the way through (it did). Using Nike + today was frustrating, it made me want a more secure/ better way of run tracking. Excited (to have a new toy to play with). (Lou, diary entry, 29, F)

Users' feelings of completion related to capturing their practices, as well as achieving set goals, were often peppered with simultaneous relief and anxiety over whether the application would work effectively and a concern that this would affect their activity. This research data supports existing literature, which exposes the inaccuracies of these devices and the data collected, particularly around partial or incomplete recordings (Beer, 2009; Mort and Smith, 2009; Cheney-Lippold, 2011; Ruppert, 2011; boyd and Crawford, 2012; Lupton, 2013b). Consistency in capturing data with every run, workout or meal was a real concern because, if effective, this led to an accumulative data trail, lifelogging and a self-tracked representation of activity. However, it is important to recognise that these findings do not advocate a utopian data double but rather a fabricated and carefully curated construction. This was often indirectly due to the variable efficacy and precision of the applications or devices (Van Remoortel et al, 2012; Lupton, 2013a, 2013b). Users were frequently frustrated when the technology did not efficiently track distances due to the failure of the application itself or the device battery, which undermined its credibility:

> I couldn't use my tracking app as I was in a rush, and it was taking particularly long to load prior to my ride. If I had waited for it to load, I was afraid that I was going to miss my train. I didn't want to give up an extra 2 minutes in bed, so I can have 2 minutes fiddling on my phone (…) Whereas before when I had a stopwatch, I'd go in and 'click' 'click. (Fred, diary entry, 30, M)

Anxiety around the fallibility of the apps was a frequent cause for worry for users and they often mentioned their unreliability (Mol, 2009). As mentioned earlier, frustrations related to the 'real' or offline world (stopping at a pedestrian crossing, for example) affected the overall statistics within the users' set goals, tending to produce emotionally embodied pressures. The fallibility of the apps, when data is lost or incorrectly captured, is a real concern for self-trackers. Reliance on the correct and continual visualisation of data provided the participants with gratifying evidence of their physical accomplishments (Ruckenstein, 2017), demonstrating their reliance on data capture of physical activity. These users' perspective supports Rettberg's (2018: 29) argument that 'we may even trust our devices more than our own experience'. Similarly, applications and devices were often considered not very user friendly (Oudshoorn, 2011). Some users find that 'getting to know' their device or application was disruptive of their existing practices.

Avoiding 'obsessive' health performativity

These pervasive considerations to and continual representations of 'health' meant that over time many self-trackers became concerned about being perceived online and offline as (explained in their own words) an 'obsessive health freak'. In terms of practices and behaviours, this was interpreted as an individual who only ever ate 'healthy foods' such as vegetables or salad and exercised rigorously. This included personality and identity traits associated with being a strict, self-regulatory and inflexible person, lacking in spontaneity and excitement in their life(style). Not being perceived as 'obsessive' about managing health, then, was an ongoing consideration for users and disciples of health. In turn, users employed careful representational strategies to avoid this. For example, constructions of this 'healthy self' were enabled through careful inclusion and exclusion of certain health information (Kent, 2020). As Sophie stated:

> 'I would post something a bit unhealthy *just* so I don't look like I'm completely obsessive. Felt pleased that I was uploading a bit more of a wholesome looking meal as I was conscious that most of my recent posts on the page were of green veg arranged on a plate.' (Sophie, final interview, 31, F)

Sophie posted the image of her 'cheat' meal on a day she was going for a run (Figure 5.1). This post was shared in an attempt to contradict or challenge any perceived 'imagined' judgement from her social media

Figure 5.1: Sophie's 'cheat' meal

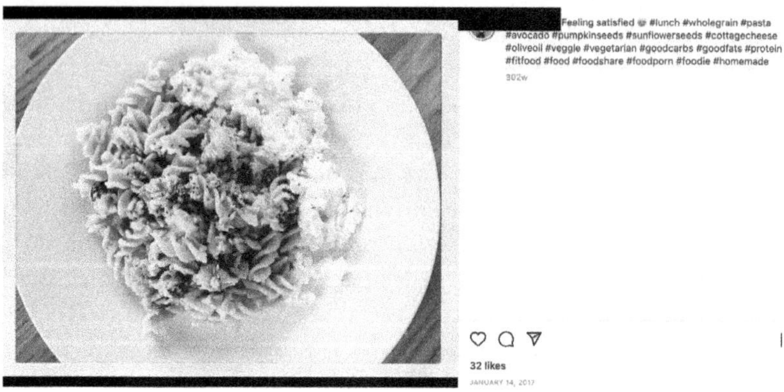

community (in this case Instagram) of her obsessively eating and posting only 'healthy' foods. The opportunity to post something other than vegetables on this user's Instagram was relished in order to diminish or avoid representations of being an 'obsessive health freak'. What is striking about this meal is that it has healthy ingredients, and it is interesting that she mentions #goodfats. It is as though the cheat meal must conform to the notion of healthiness, whereby the discipline of being and performing the digital health self must be consistently represented even when attempts at 'authenticity' mean sharing 'less healthy' foods; many would still perceive these as containing nutritious and not unhealthy ingredients. Representation of the digital healthy self still prevails as conforming to diet culture discourse and norms.

This also demonstrates how imagined audiences and the community (Anderson, 1983) online are maintained through the carefully balanced mediation between self-censorship and exposure, through an 'ongoing loop of impression management mixed and based upon audience feedback' (Marwick and boyd, 2010: 13). This 'impression management', however, cannot always be maintained through content that represents specific and different 'health' identities. The participants' attempts at avoiding representations of being an 'obsessive health freak' were at times scuppered as these foods were frequently identified as not 'Instagram-worthy(sic)' or 'Instagrammable(sic)' (Sophie, 31, final interview). They were therefore concealed and not uploaded, as they were seen as 'unattractive':

> 'Last night I made Thai Red Curry and I thought "oh, that looks a bit better" because sometimes I think it is just salad, but then sometimes I make more wholesome stuff, but it just doesn't look as pretty so then I can't post it. If I've spent ages making food and it's really tasty and then I go to take a picture and it just looked bad I'm like "oh I can't post it after all that faffing around". I couldn't post my breakfast this morning, it really irritated me.' (Sophie, final interview, 31, F)

More analysis of meal curation is covered in Chapter 6; however, here we can see the practices of preparing, capturing and sharing 'health' self-representations, in particular food and meals, are labour-intensive and time-consuming processes, which convey an attempt to appear 'in the moment'. This individualistic striving for perfection is best understood as entrepreneurial self-work and, more specifically, self-capitalisation concentrated on the visual register (Conor, 2004), effected through consumer regimes of beauty (Gill, 2007b). This premeditated curation is deemed 'worth it' only when enough likes or positive feedback is received from the community, which can be achieved only when images are 'pretty' enough to post. Users also experienced frustration when misrepresentations of health identity are perceived in offline settings. As Lou explained when she felt concerned about how her peers judged her eating habits:

> 'I've been trying to relax my attitude towards food but it's hard when I eat around people as I feel they are judging, but I feel like I am probably to blame for posting all of the healthy pics in the first place as then I feel I need to live up to it. I bumped into a friend at the train station the other day who was ordering a bacon roll and she commented how I wouldn't approve and jokingly apologised. I know she wasn't being really serious, but it did make me think about how I come across to people.' (Lou, final interview, 29, F)

'Living' up to the expectations of others within online and offline spheres was a concern for all the participants (as examined throughout this book). Poor body image, as perceived by others, affected how users perceived themselves (Cederstrom and Spicer, 2015). Therefore, online (and offline) feedback operates in this context bubble of idealised bodies, diets and lifestyles. Interestingly, these 'poor' perceptions were not just in relation to being perceived as 'unhealthy' or as suffering from an eating disorder. Rather, being 'obsessive' was defined as being over-regulatory and overtly controlling of the self, which was not positively regarded by the broader online community. For many users, attempts at 'truth telling' were delivered with consideration of community norms (for example, avoiding representations of obsessive 'healthy' lifestyles by posting a 'cheat meal'), ensuring that a careful representation of an authentic 'digital health self' was constructed. Ironically, in pursuing the appearance of authenticity for the gaze of others, users ended up constructing an arguably inauthentic representation of self (Kent, 2020). These findings challenge the dominant discourses of 'sharing' and confessional cultures (Beer, 2010), as evidenced by social media usage, since it can be clearly identified that such practices have shifted, as users age with and alongside these platforms. These findings contribute to a more critical form of engagement with such technologies, centring around questions related to the use of data (Beer, 2016), surveillance and coercive powers (Lupton, 2014b; Andrejevic, 2015). It is worth mentioning that the changes to the European Union's General Data Protection Regulation (GDPR, eugdpr.org) in 2018, and the Cambridge Analytica data mining scandal whereby up to 87 million people had their Facebook data scraped by the political consultancy (Wired.co.uk, 10/4/18), may have to an extent increased public awareness of how data, privacy and surveillance operated in daily use of these platforms, as well as for future mining. Other popular culture documentaries such as 'The Great Hack' (Dir. Karim Amer and Jehane Noujaim, 2019), 'The Social Dilemma' (Dir. Jeff Orlowski, 2020) and 'Coded Bias' (Dir. Shalini

Kantayya, 2020) have arguably contributed to broader public awareness of data mining and a loss of privacy as an ideological trade-off for using digital platforms and services. However, it is worth noting that awareness does not always translate to comprehensive understanding in everyday uses of these platforms' privacy policies from a user perspective. Loss of privacy of personal data arguably continues to be the often-accepted trade-off for using free digital platforms.

From social media use and compulsion to 'addiction'

The chapters until now have identified the many habitual practices and processes related to social media and self-tracking platforms from the perspectives of those who use these platforms extensively for sharing and surveilling health practices in their everyday lives. Over time, increasing and habitual use of both social media platforms and health apps became identified by users as 'compulsive'. The 'compulsion' to use these platforms to manage health also includes the habitual surveillance of others' health practices within these networks. In recent years, compulsion and 'addiction' towards technology, in particular social media, have become increasingly addressed by psychiatric research and now by many academic disciplines including internet and digital media scholars. Given its increasing 'buzzword' status, it is worth pausing here, before analysing the empirical data, for a definition of technology and social media 'addiction'.

'Addiction' to social media tends to refer to compulsions towards its use and its negative impacts on wellbeing (Lupton, 2016). Psychiatric research identifies social media addiction as a specific form of technology addiction (American Psychiatric Association, 2013), which manifests itself in

> addiction-like symptoms, including salience (preoccupation with the behaviour), mood modification (performing the behaviour to relieve or reduce aversive emotional states), tolerance (increasing engagement in the behaviour over time to attain the initial mood modifying effects), withdrawal (experiencing psychological and physical discomfort when the behaviour is reduced or prohibited), conflict (putting off or neglecting social, recreational, work, educational, household and/ or other activities as well as one's own and others' needs because of the behaviour), and relapse (unsuccessfully attempting to cut down or control the behaviour). (He et al, 2017a: 84)

This chapter does not attempt to determine in psychiatric terms whether social media 'addiction' should be an established clinical classification (He et al, 2017b). However, what is of importance is examining the impact and characteristics of these addictive and compulsive traits upon participants' everyday lives and how these symptoms were in many respects similar to established 'addictions' (Dong et al, 2012). In relation to the participants' use of social media, the traits of addictive behaviours as outlined in the aforementioned extract by He et al (2017b) were exhibited by all the participants during my research study. Interestingly, some participants described themselves as having addictive tendencies towards social media. Furthermore, those that did not refer to themselves as social media 'addicts' did indeed demonstrate some 'addictive' behaviours in relation to platform use and expressed compulsive desires towards their devices. For example, sharing all aspects of their life, even regarding activities unrelated to health, became an everyday priority:

> 'In my head, whenever I was doing anything, I was thinking (…) "what can I share online?" (…) I was just obsessed. I can't go down the beach without getting a picture, what's the point? Every single thing that I was doing, even if it wasn't to do with fitness, if there was an occasion I was thinking already in my head: "oh, brilliant opportunity, how am I going to put this on social media."' (Sophie, final interview, 31, F)

Frequently, the impulse to simply share for sharing's sake becomes for many users a daily occurrence, which can evolve into an increasingly inherent desire to divulge all aspects of their lives on social media. Users can become 'overly concerned about social media activities, driven by an uncontrollable motivation to perform the behaviour' (Dong and Potenza, 2014: np) Being invited to an event or making plans socially or professionally provided participants with a gratifying sense of life being busy and social and contributing to a form of status and identity as social middle-class professionals in contemporary digital capitalism (Wajcman, 2014). To extend Wajcman's (2014) argument, social media (and converged self-tracking technologies) enabled participants with a representational outlet to perform such identities. However, what was of particular interest was that alongside the ability for performative self-representation was the participants' sense of elation in knowing such 'events' enabled opportunities to capture a busy social life and to then share these self-representations on social media. Bizarrely, the gratification from posting at times became the dominant focus and motivation for these participants to attend events, socialise and undertake certain activities, demonstrating the normative and naturalised embedding of these technologies of the self and their interference in participants' everyday lives (Dong and Potenza, 2014). In turn, the representation of an idealised online life captured and shared on social media motivated the offline and lived experiences of these health disciples.

The significance of this curated online representation directly forming and moulding offline experience was exemplified prominently during exercise regimes:

> 'I think it had just become such a thing that I was running and I would take a photo when I saw something interesting and then I'd post it and be like "hey look what I've done this morning" and I was like "oh god, I haven't seen anything interesting and I'm almost at the end. It's going to have to be a picture of my shoe." I was like "no, you're not running to get a picture, you're running to get the distance that you've done. You're just going to have to not post anything today." It just became a bit ridiculous. I was freaking out, not over the fact that I've not run far enough, more that I'm nearly home and I've not got a picture. I think that made me reassess what I was doing, it shouldn't make you that stressed.' (Lou, final interview, 29, F)

Here Lou reflects in her final interview that, whilst marathon training, she became extremely concerned and 'stressed' about capturing a scenic representation of her training runs. For example, if a run was not picturesque in a way users could share on social media, this sometimes compels them to keep running or exercising so they can find a more visually attractive location to photograph and then share. If not, they frequently express anxiety that they cannot document their health efforts in a way their social media community would deem interesting or aesthetically pleasing. Thus, although training or exercising goals might be met, the lack of representation of this interferes with self-trackers' sense of pleasure and gratification gained from running (Dong and Potenza, 2014). This tension was similarly demonstrated by Sophie when trying to capture her physical muscular growth and 'gains' from boxing in the gym:

> At the gym I asked the guys I was training with to take pictures for my Instagram. One took some really bad pictures and I got really frustrated at him. I was just really horrible, in my head I thought I'm going to get this amazing picture to post. I'd done all this boxing, I felt good, amazing progress. That was the first time I had started to notice some of my gains in my back and shoulders, thinking 'wow it would be cool if I can post a picture of that'. Afterwards I felt really bad for being rude to him. (Sophie, diary entry, 31, F)

In both these examples, running or exercising can be wholly motivated by the desire to want to get a photographic representation, which can then be shared on social media. Here we can see the illustration of Turel et al's (2017) argument that compulsions towards social media can be exemplified by an uncontrollable motivation to perform that behaviour. This often replaced users' sense of emotional fulfilment from achieving personal goals. Sophie was irritated by her friend who did not capture an appealing image of her muscle 'gains' in the gym. Lou became annoyed when she could not capture a pretty landscape during her marathon training runs. Although users might recognise these frustrations as 'ridiculous' and 'distracting them' from the purpose of why they were exercising, these visual defeats become a genuine source and sense of personal disappointment. This demonstrates how we can conceive of these compulsive and arguably 'addictive' behaviours as harmful when users cannot stop enacting them despite their ability to see their negative impacts (Alter, 2017).

The choice architecture of attention

For these users, compulsions frequently focused towards capturing the 'perfect' image of the healthy, fit self and they were satisfied when such representations were achieved. For example, Sophie spent hours in the gym trying to capture a 'good' image after the first (poor) attempt. When eventually satisfied with the 'ideal' representation of her body, she posted it on Facebook and Instagram (Figure 5.2). This demonstrated how time estimates, compulsive behaviour, overuse and tolerance became justified through personal bias (Rau et al, 2006; Lin et al, 2015) towards achieving representational goals and in this case the 'perfect image':

> I feel great after posting the picture. I've had positive comments on Facebook and lots of likes on Instagram. I feel like checking the comments and how many likes I've had has taken over the whole evening though. It's addictive checking how many people have liked the picture. It's nice to see people who don't usually bother liking my 'selfie' pictures liking this picture. It's like they take it and me more seriously. (Sophie, diary entry, 31, F)

For many users (and Sophie is not alone), numerous hours were dedicated to photographing self-improvement, for example, muscle 'gains' in the gym or 'before and after' photos of weight loss, sharing it on social media and checking the feedback from the community. A sharer of a wide variety of different health-related content (fitness selfies, food photography and self-tracking data), Sophie was very aware of who in her online network usually 'liked' certain content. This inverted panoptic gaze (Lupton, 2012b) (the surveillance of the community surveying her) on this post provided Sophie with additional gratification that those who usually 'like' or comment on data sharing (as recognised in the previous section) for its valued legitimacy also 'liked' this image. This contributed to her sense of identity as a 'serious' 'healthy' role model and influencer on social media. It is, therefore, very important for users

Figure 5.2: Sophie's 'muscle gains' post

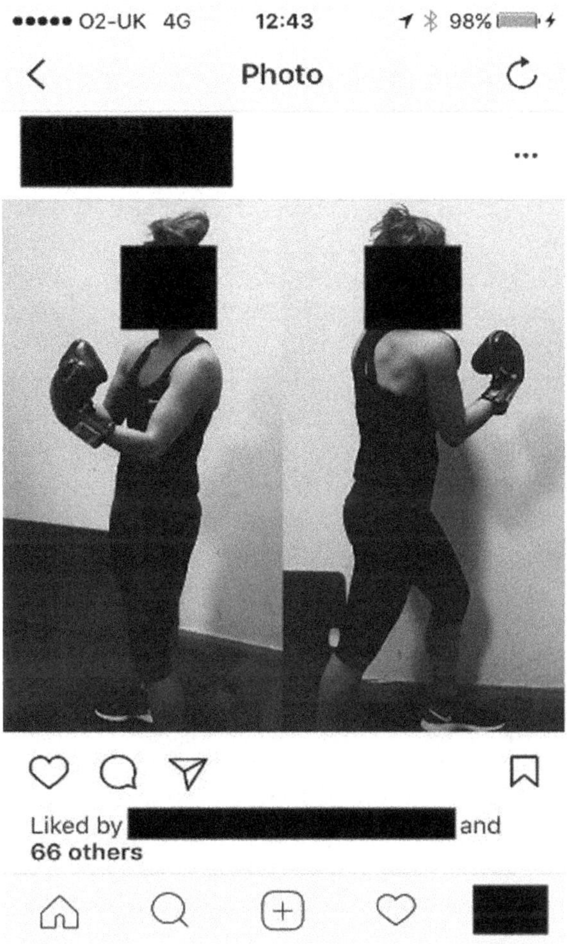

that their communities' perceptions were influenced and managed through these carefully constructed self-representations of 'healthy' bodies. However, checking 'likes' and feedback from the community to determine if the post had been positively and 'correctly' received took up huge amounts of the participants' time, often distracting them from their everyday lives such as dominating an evening intended for relaxing (in Sophie's example).

Behavioural 'addictions' exacerbated through technology

Behavioural 'addictions' arise when a person can't resist a behaviour that, despite addressing a deep psychological need in the short term, produces significant harm in the long term (Alter, 2017). This is exemplified problematically in the following participant extract:

> My phone's just glued to my hands every night. Like, last night I was just checking my phone, how many likes have I got, just checking. it's weird. Why does it matter if you get loads of 'likes', but you feel good or if you don't get hardly any [you don't feel good]? It's hard to explain, but it just becomes obsessive. (Sophie, diary entry, 31, F)

To refer to an attachment to a device as 'glued' to your physical body shows the deep mental and physical connection to it, such that it is difficult to be without the device. Alter (2017: np) argues that neoliberal societies hold an expectation of convenience, which has 'weaponised temptation'. It is arguable that the behavioural economic structures of gamification in social media and digital health platforms can not only hugely impact behavioural change but also create 'addiction' type symptoms. It is worth reiterating that the techno-commercial infrastructures of these digital platforms draw upon UX (user experience) designs within behavioural economics, prioritising the metrics of the attention economy in generating value for these businesses. If the 'attention economy' (Simon, 1970) is 'a state in which cognitive resources are focused on certain aspects of the environment rather than on others' (American Psychological Association, 2020), then the value of the attention economy on social media and health apps is the metrics of engagement: the likes, shares, posts, follows and comments, as well as products and services advertised on the platforms themselves. Arguably, the function of the app, whether for social or health purposes, is largely irrelevant to commercial interest, so long as it is being increasingly used by an ever-expanding user base. The monetisation of attention in the digital economy under platform capitalism is the goal of the developers of these applications, along with the increasing enmeshment of these tools in users' everyday lives. Of course, to be used, an application must be relevant, with enticing user experience to ensure the app is commercially viable to maintain.

The behavioural economics of gamification design strategies arguably come in very useful to generate and create 'addiction like' practices in self-tracking users over time; 'the system (logically or not) [is] easier to use and better in serving the [user's] intrinsic and extrinsic needs' (Turel et al, 2011: 1049). This 'system' is designed by a 'choice architect' who Thaler and Sunstein (2009: 3) argue has the 'the responsibility for organizing the context in which people make decisions'. This argument is based upon an oversimplifying (and rather arrogant) assumption that when it comes to decision-making choice architects know better than individuals and thus orchestrate an environment to influence such behaviour or decisions for them. This is achieved through design nudges, for example, a notification for a 'like' on social media platforms or an exercise reminder on a health app; indeed it 'is any aspect of the choice architecture that alters people's behavior in a predictable way without forbidding any options or significantly changing their economic incentives' (Thaler and Sunstein, 2009: 6). Arguably 'addiction' and gamification are most useful in the context of healthcare applications in creating a healthier lifestyle, complementing long-term behavioural change; however, in time, this can have extremely adverse effects in over-exertion and injury. Arguments for the moral underpinning of the gamification of healthcare application usually follow the discourse of creating 'healthier lifestyles', without attending to the long-term mental or physical health implications of this, such as over-exercise, injury, stress or anxiety, and tech 'addiction' induced by these problematic relationships with these companionship technologies. Furthermore, it is important to recognise that these devices cannot always take into consideration the unquantifiable, the individual emotional wellbeing, physical stress or trauma, during their data capture.

Tools of temptation

The empirical data presented throughout this book, and particularly in this chapter, illustrates how the techno-commercial platform infrastructures of Facebook, Instagram and some health apps are seen by many users as tools of temptation, embedded with a deep attachment to practices that are also sometimes compulsive and difficult to stop. Users cannot often identify why the habitual nature of checking their phones was such a pervasive compulsive behaviour in their everyday lives and cannot always see through the obstructive marketing veil of normalising platform and surveillance capitalism. If we were to (rather reductively) set aside the commercial infrastructure of platform design, choice architecture and behavioural economics in this influential dynamic, we can extend the conversation with users about how to explain their attachment and connection to their devices.

What these platforms of companionship do for users, arguably, is provide a lens of perspective via data acquisition, particularly with regard to personal health and biometric statistics. These perspectives provide certain ways of knowing what data is, why it is important, who gets to interpret it and to what ends. As Ajana (2013: 10) asserts: 'citizenship is seen as becoming a hollowed out concept whose carcass is increasingly shaped around techniques of identity management.' These technologies, over time, through a long term relationship with data acquisition become 'addictive companions' and extensions of our physicality, attached to our being whilst emotionally and technologically mediating our everyday lives and individual identities. Regardless of not knowing *why* they returned to check feedback, users continue to be seduced by the socio-technological affordances of social media and digital health tools. The Medical Futurist (2017: np) argue that this comes down to the focus on change: 'Motivation is one factor in changing behaviour, but loyalty towards the subject of change is something people usually don't consider.' This loyalty to change is exemplified through some metrics of status and sociality within these platforms and data-sharing social media spheres. For example, the currency of acquiring 'likes' provides an intangible yet emotional value and contribution to users' sense of self. Similarly, the surveillance of others' similar practices via social media provides a sense of comradery: a unified community of health-orientated individuals working towards changing their lives through healthy living. However, when surveying and 'scrolling' similar accounts become a regular practice over time, it can contribute to distracting users from personal goals:

> I did get distracted by yoga photos on Instagram- still haven't done any yoga as a result of scrolling. Feel I need to put boundaries on my time on that too, or give myself a rule, that if something inspires me, to take action instead of continuing to scroll. I've deleted Facebook from my phone to save myself from distraction. (Lara, diary entry, 28, F)

> 'I do get the aimless scrolling thing. Sometimes I get locked into it.' (Annie, final interview, 28, F)

Scrolling on social media can cause some impairment in other life domains for self-tracking users. In these examples, it diverted users' attention from doing their own exercise. Similar to documenting and sharing, scanning through health-related content draws users into a compulsive surveillant practice. The obsessive yet mesmerising practice of surveillance of others held within its own process the same compulsive traits of documenting and sharing the participants' own lives. As Alter (2017: 33) argues, 'Addictions bring the promise of immediate rewards, or positive reinforcement. In contrast, obsessions and compulsions are intensely unpleasant to not pursue. They promise relief (…) but not the appealing rewards of a consummated addiction.' Often, users feel the only way to reject the 'addictive hold' these practices had over their lives was to detox from social media, by either deleting the application for a period of time or quitting it altogether.

Digital detoxing and quitting social media

Digital detox describes efforts to take a break from online or digital media for a longer or shorter period, as well as other efforts to restrict the use of smartphones and digital tools (Kent, 2020). Digital detox is a phenomenon that presents a promise of authenticity, set within a presumption that mediated interactions or time spent on digital platforms or without face-to-face communication is inauthentic (Syvesten and Enli, 2020). In addition to describing a set of practices, digital detox appears in books, blogs, websites and social media posts as a buzzword, representing certain understandings of the pervasive role of digital media in everyday life. Buzzwords, in popular culture and news media, are created to simplify complex practices and relations signalling newness, legitimating and proposing a strategy of intervention (Mjøs et al, 2014). Unlike many buzzwords in the digital society of today, which are often celebrating digital technology's intervention in our everyday life, this one takes a dystopian lens on technology and looks nostalgically to a time when life was not so intensely mediated, technology was less intrusive and we had more time uninterrupted by technology (Enli, 2015). This final section of the chapter will examine the reasons behind shifting social media practices over time, in consideration of increasing moves towards digital detoxing and decisions of some users to quit altogether.

Digital detox draws on a variety of inspirations and motivations. Digital detox also draws upon Buddhist notions of mindfulness, spirituality and balance, which have been widely co-opted and repacked by a now highly lucrative international wellness industry (Syvesten and Enli, 2020). Corporate self-optimisation through wellness schemes encourages improving productivity by reducing digital distractions (Guyard and Kaun, 2018; Till, 2018). Most interestingly perhaps, mindfulness is now often promoted through a lens of self-regulation and self-discipline for improving one's thoughts and emotions to overcome daily stresses (Glomb et al, 2011: 123). Digital detox is frequently presented by the wellness industry and corporate wellness schemes as a solution to enhance employees' performance, achieve a balanced life and improve mental health. Other examples of the digital detox discourse exist in consumer activism and institutional resistance against potential negative media effects (Syvesten and Enli, 2020).

Media history has presented many opportunities for cultural moral panic before in relation to the fear of technological overload (Cohen, 1985; Williams, 1981). For example, in the sixteenth century, 'the multitude of books' prompted warnings that literary overload could lead to a 'barbarous' future unless effective reading strategies were adopted to manage the overwhelming influx of material (Blair, 2003: 11; in Syvesten and Enli, 2020: x). Fast forward to the 1980s and the wide adoption of television in the home prompted a political and media outbreak of panic similarly associated with its detrimental disruption upon and invasion of precious family time (Williams, 1981). Wajcman (2014; 2) contends that today the 'iconic image that abounds is that of the frenetic, technologically tethered, iPhone-or-iPad-addicted citizen', and thus what we can argue for today's moral panic is that non-mediated time is disappearing in daily life. The 'accessible anytime, anywhere' culture is heavily subscribed to around the world by those that are connected (Lomborg, 2011; 36). In this vein, digital detox presents an opportunity for detachment from our heavily mediated digital lives.

Motivations to digitally detox

Fundamentally, we can see digital detox as one of the latest iterations of neoliberalism, denoting individual responsibility to resist overload from technology, reflected extensively in the empirical data presented in this book. For users, this becomes particularly hard to enact but increasingly necessary when life became busy or stressful:

> I haven't posted a lot recently. I have been quite stressed out with a few conflicts at home and been having a bit of a break from people and social media. We managed to secure a flat the other day. Yet the next day I was made redundant. Although it hasn't affected my training, my diet has been terrible, therefore I have not posted much. (Annie, diary entry, 28, F)

A 'break' from social media often became imperative when personal and professional lives were overwhelming. The motivation to detach was twofold. Firstly, when individual lives were stressful, this often took time away from being able to enact healthy behaviours, for example, eating well and going to the gym, as detailed by Annie. Secondly, when personal and/or professional life was demanding and overwhelming users felt they could not contribute to idealised representations of 'healthy' lives or view others doing so on social media, as this contributed to feelings of comparative anxiety, inadequacy and personal disempowerment, which negatively impacted their sense of 'health self' and identity as a disciple of health:

> 'At the beginning of this year, I had a bit of a breakdown and just couldn't really cope with anything, so I've come off social media, I just don't want to feel the pressure to prove to everyone what my life is like or spend all my energy lifting everyone else up. I've just got to the point where I need to concentrate on myself. I thought trying to save everyone else would in turn save me and lift me up but actually it just fully drained me, and I've had to step back.' (Annie, final interview, 28, F)

> I felt that my daily commute is stressful enough to add another thing to it. I know it was only a weekly progress, but on Mondays I knew I was going to share after my commute, I just felt 'enough', I no longer wanted to be burdened by it. (Fet, diary entry, 30, M)

Over long periods of time, continually posting and updating their online communities about their lives create an emotional pressure for users. Not posting can be seen as indicative of enabling privacy, needing personal time and space away from social media, especially during life's challenging times. Interestingly, the language articulated in these quotes from Fet and Annie demonstrates a discourse of social media providing a tangible emotional space in their everyday lives and routines, one which can be stepped away from. Therefore, although exhibiting a different motivation than is discussed in Chapter 6, the concealment of 'unhealthy' behaviours to avoid judgement from others in this case similarly relieves users from being the object of their communities' gaze and judging their own lives by comparing lifestyles represented and viewed on social media. In this space, users continuously affirm each other through sharing and liking, and in turn these practices of affirmation not only are visible to others but build trust and community (Thiel-Stern, 2012; Schreiber and Kramer, 2016). For many users, filling the void with social media (Gilroy-Ware, 2017) meant that when they reflected upon these habits they realised how much they had been drawn into consuming 'addictive' and habitual self-regulatory cycles of self-tracking, monitoring the self and sharing these behaviours with their communities.

Co-evolving with social media sharing

> 'If you looked at social media usage pre-relationship ending and then post-relationship ending, it's gone up hundreds of percent, I threw myself into it.' (Sophie, final interview, 31, F)

Changes in personal lives, circumstances and mental health influence users' social media sharing and health practices. One participant, Annie, described social media detachment as 'coming away from it' both physically and emotionally. When users chose not to share or not to use certain platforms, or wanted a 'digital detox', social media platforms were spaces that had to be physically stepped away from, thus highlighting the pervasiveness of its inbuilt interpersonal surveillance (Trottier, 2012) and its dominant role in their daily lives. Digital detoxing is usually identified by users as a significant challenge, for the benefit of mental health, but also as something that was an internal negotiation and often an internal contention pulling some users' 'addictive' compulsions towards it. Because of the habitual use of social media, its 'addictive nature' was experienced similarly to a drug and with it followed a similar discourse to describe abstinence, 'giving up', 'quitting' or going 'cold turkey'. This resistance to technology was achieved for some users by framing the detachment in medical terms. Quitting 'just because' was not a discourse, and often medical language legitimated the decision to 'detox'.

> 'Now with Facebook's application of "memories" (…) I find myself anxiously thinking I shared loads about everything.' (Fet, final interview, 30, M)

> 'I used to always post on Facebook and now I barely put anything up, I think Instagram is just a newer fad. I think it will get boring or something else will come along. I don't think I've had any moments where it's some sort of epiphany, like "that's it, I'm off social media, I don't need to prove myself anymore". There's obviously still a bit of me inside, I still think I need to do this sometimes but I think it has made me reassess what I post and why, because you know you go through those phases of seeing people like "this is my hairstyle today" and I'm like "I don't care". I don't ever want to be that person where someone looks at my post and thinks "for god's sake".' (Lara, final interview, 28, F)

In this quote, Lara discusses broader trends and social media etiquettes. For example, seeing others 'oversharing' makes users paranoid and aware of how they are perceived, which can encourage participants to detox from their digital devices. Sharing etiquettes develop by seeing others oversharing, which prompts a consciousness that one does not want to be perceived in that way by others in the online community. In turn, this encourages online silence. The Facebook 'memories' function nudges and prompts users to view content they shared on certain days of using the platform over the years (since they joined); this can remind users of content previously shared that, as they co-evolve with the technology, they now deem to be 'oversharing'. These previous (over)sharing practices can cause shame and embarrassment in the present day. These examples highlight shifting social media sharing practices and cultures, which develop and emerge with the co-evolving process of aging alongside and along with social media platforms.

We have a right to disconnect and to interrupt networks, but we still hold on to other versions of the social (actual and imaginary). We could then consider that social media networks (and the widespread disciplinary systems in which they are embedded) are an explicit attempt to construct social media and related interpersonal surveillance until it seems natural and as though we cannot imagine our social lives or communicative practices without it. This perspective is reflected in Lou's words, when she draws together the emotionally embodied pressure to engage with these platforms and technology to gain connectedness online, which became such a normalised process it distracted her from her personal experience:

> 'That was probably one of the posts where I was like "you don't need to take a picture every time. What you're actually doing is training for a marathon, not proving that marathon training to other people, you will prove that training when you finish it. That's your goal, not 'likes' on social networks. Just stop being an idiot."' (Lou, final interview, 29, F)

> I felt the need to stop sharing because I was getting more and more drawn into my devices and social media platform for something that I already knew; that I was improving with my cycling during my commute. (Fet, diary entry, 30, M)

Many users try to resist their own (what had become) normalised practice of regular sharing on social media (van Dijck, 2014) and recognise when the pressure to document shifted focus away from actual exercise. Those who did 'detox' from social media were motivated to do so as they felt their social media use was damaging their mental health but struggled with abstaining due to their previous habitual use. Social media sharing shifted over time in line with the participants' changing lives. Being a consistent inspirational figure to others on social media by constantly sharing and documenting one's life became an oppressive pressure. The continual self-regulation needed to self-track, capture, document and share became an exhausting process for all participants at some point during the research period. Interestingly, even though they recognised that all social media and self-tracking users must feel this way, those that did detox or quit embodied feelings of being unique. For example, one participant considered himself 'different' and resisting conformity by quitting social media:

> 'By not sharing I have that power back with me, that I don't succumb to the norm I guess.' (Fet, final interview, 30, M)

Therefore, the social media norms within these communities perpetuate the idea that sharing is the common practice and not sharing is the deviant or unusual behaviour. A sense of empowerment is achieved by resisting and quitting these persuasive and coercive technologies of health management (Purpura et al, 2011). The self, therefore, feels liberated from overt disciplinary and regulatory control over personal health through technology and surveillance. From a longitudinal perspective, these sentiments were echoed by most of the participants in this research. Looking to the future, all participants saw themselves continuing with their 'health' and fitness practices but were unsure if they would use self-tracking devices to capture these practices or social media to document them. Those who were detoxing or had quit did in fact see themselves returning in the future. Interestingly, this was due to feelings guilt because of neglect towards the devices and platforms, as well as their online communities:

> 'I still feel guilt sometimes (…) If I do post, nothing really gets commented on but when I used to do it tonnes of people would tune in. I feel like I've let people down. I still beat myself up when I think about it. I should've been stronger. I should've kept going. I know

> that one day when I'm in a better place I can go back and build up again and then it's another story isn't it. I miss showing people what a fun life you can have, what fun I have and just sharing. I have started making YouTube videos actually. Rather than putting pressure on myself every day, I'll film something and every two or three weeks I'll post (…) that's one way of getting something out. But it's weird because my whole life revolved around social media for so long.' (Annie, final interview, 28, F)

Interestingly, users who felt that they missed sharing their lives online and missed their social media communities often felt a responsibility towards them. Time offline enables certain mental headspace and reduction in feelings of anxiety around pressures to post. Over time, this can develop into feelings of withdrawal, which often manifests as guilt due to a lack of contact with their community or health and fitness developments, or FOMO ('fear of missing out'), for many users. This withdrawal often then manifested into feelings of being responsible for keeping others online updated about individual life events ('health'-related or not). As identified in earlier chapters, expectation to share within the community was an embodied pressure. Yet the user examples in this chapter highlight how these feelings are still prevalent, even when social media or self-tracking is identified as being detrimental to users' mental health. Guilt associated with not sharing is not (as one might expect) diminished even though there is realisation that using these technologies, tracking and sharing negatively affects one's sense of self.

Conclusions

In the digital society of today, the 'health disciple' is focused on developing many different attributes to extensively manage their healthcare. This frequently asserts itself with the individual striving to seek out health, fitness and wellbeing information for everyday optimal health management. I conceptualise this health self-practice as becoming a 'lay expert' of health, which over time can develop into self-policing practices. The self-policing can grow into compulsive or even arguably 'addictive' behaviours over time; this is due to a number of factors including the pressures of community visibility and surveillance as well as the behavioural economics and 'nudging' infrastructure of social media and health apps reminding users to engage, share and perform their discipline to health. These regulatory and compulsive self and community surveillance practices have led many users to detox digitally, abstaining for a period of time or quitting altogether.

Over time, individuals who had quit temporarily or permanently still identified feelings of responsibility to self-track their behaviours and a commitment to social media to share their lives, highlighting the dominance of these platforms' integration into their sense of self, their 'health' identity and their use in everyday life. This chapter explored the compulsive and addictive practices and shifting behaviours over time through the discourse of a 'health disciple', which is a defining characteristic of 'the health self' mantra in users' everyday life. Aside from these worrying traits and behaviours, what is also worth noting, from the perspective of the social sciences, psychiatry and the medical humanities, is the challenge of identifying the boundaries that constitute such 'addictions' (Turel et al, 2011). Another challenge for researchers is that the appropriate language and clinical terminology used to describe these behaviours and neuro-physiological states are not yet agreed upon (Lortie and Guitton, 2013). The distinction between an 'addiction' (the indulgence of which brings pleasure) and a compulsion (the indulgence of which merely brings relief from restless anxiety) (Alter, 2017) blurs linguistic and psychiatric boundaries with these technologies. In digitised societies, it is culturally assumed and almost expected that most users compulsively check their devices and social media. These practices challenge a once-dominant cultural discourse, which assumed that social media usage offered a break from boredom or a habitual distraction tool. In practice, this behaviour became a habit and a compulsion in which participants took their time in deciding how to detox or quit. These technologies, however, hold 'addictive', persuasive and influential power over our lives, for even when we resist them, we still feel a duty towards their use and integration into our everyday lives. This most interestingly, and alarmingly, highlights the pervasively 'addictive' cycle of our relationship with technology: salience, mood modification, tolerance, withdrawal, conflict and relapse. In turn, we can see how tech 'addiction' could now align with and be illustrative of established clinical 'addictive traits and behaviours'.

This is why it is important to recognise that when digital detox is presented as the solution, this places pressure on individual responsibility and not enough agency on platform capitalism. This over-emphasis on digital detox being attainable a level of individual responsibility, is not only hard to implement in daily life living in the digital society of today but additionally does not take into consideration techno-commercial affordances, choice architecture or the relentless 'nudges' of devices. Digital health and social media practices are arguably 'addictive' due to the choice architecture of platform capitalism; these platforms are built to keep our attention. Therefore, these findings contradict Nafus and Neff's (2016) proposition that many self-trackers use data to create new habits or stop or change existing ones, when in fact this analysis identified that not only did these pervasive digital technologies provoke and reinforce existing habits, for example excessive exercise, calorie counting or over-analysis and evaluation of the body (image), but they also stoked anxieties and created new habits that are often detrimental to users' mental and physical health and wellbeing. This manifested itself as users comparing themselves to others' habits, exercise routines or body (image), and an over-reliance on virtual support and gratification from feedback frequently distracts users from personal achievements and, perhaps most worryingly, personal enjoyment and experiences in their everyday lives. Even when technology was removed entirely or resisted due to perceived 'addiction' or 'compulsive use', the regulation of the body, with or without the tools and technologies, is still conceived as prevalent, preventative and self-policing in the minds of these users.

6

Sharing 'Healthiness'

Introduction

This chapter explores in great detail how self-tracking technologies and social media enable the management and representation of specific 'health(y)' lifestyles and identities. Through presentation of the empirical analysis (interviews, reflexive diaries and online content), it examines how the collaborative information produced within these data-sharing cultures changes user behaviours, understandings of the body and what is deemed as 'healthy', often in relation to others. The chapter identifies the many purposes and 'share-ability' of different digital representations of health on social media (van Dijck, 2013b; Tifentale and Manovich, 2015). Whether sharing for support, motivation or appearing authentic or avoiding oversharing, users represent many of their practices with the view to perform the 'idealised' body (Kent, 2018) and 'digital health self'. As we have explored in earlier chapters, self-definition through endless self-tracking maintains the optimisation of 'health' as the continual lifestyle goal for these individuals. This chapter highlights how health and lifestyle have become representative of this 'optimal self', through the representation of health choices and everyday wellness behaviours on social media platforms. Embodiment of this focus on maximising and optimising health is no longer a priority confined to the 'health-conscious', the quantified self movement, users of self-tracking technologies or social media influencers. This chapter identifies how the 'digital health self' is the conceptualisation of an everyday productive individual, citizen and subject, who self-regulates health as a performance through self-tracking data, conceiving the representation, and thus the curation, as a powerful force and in turn controlling the malleable physical form to attain the performance of a continually improving body, in the hope of a happier, healthier and optimal future.

> 'We are a generation of phone people, so you pick up your phone and you think "I checked everything so why am I picking it up a minute

> later". You're just so used to having your phone and checking you don't know what you're checking for sometimes. I think there's an element of, if there's a picture when you've just spent ages getting the filter right, and the hashtags, I faff, shall I put this hashtag, then you post it and sit there. I couldn't post a photo on Instagram and then just leave my phone on the side and wander downstairs, I feel like maybe people that do it, maybe I've got something missing in my life.' (Sophie, 31, first interview, F)

The 'digital health self' wants to perform via technology in everyday life. For users sharing health-related data, health becomes representative of the self, via acquiring self-tracking data and its performance in digital spaces. This performance enables the digital health self to become 'share-able' and shifts the role of health from individually managed to performatively available and visible on social media platforms. It is available for scrutiny, critique, assessment, idealisation or admiration. Sharing content on social media affords users a variety of ways to represent 'health'. It is thus important to explore the variety of content and data capture users curate in performance of the digital health self, in particular those which showcase how lifestyle choices and behaviour (corrections) (Leichter, 1997) have become ideologically and culturally demonstrative of individual 'health' states. The role of social media within these practices is to enable the 'healthy' individual to be both curator and subject. This othering of bodies, along with bio-political differentiation of one type of body and citizen from another (Ajana, 2012), is a dominant identifier (from others) discourse within the competitive and comparative strategies enabled by self-tracking devices, apps and social media platforms. This chapter examines the many different practices and performative tools users adopt to achieve the desired self-presentation and performance of 'healthy' and 'productive' bodies and selves, analysing the processes and practices embodied and adopted in curation of digital health self-identities.

This chapter's analysis draws upon Goffman's (1959: 22) definition of self-presentation as a performance, described as the 'activity of an individual which occurs during a period marked by his continuous presence before a set of observers and which has some influence on his observers'. Though written in 1959, his observations of front and back stages, I argue, draw parallels with the distinctions and paradoxes with online and offline performative divides, negotiations and navigations. Through the 'front stage' we are trying to present an idealised version of the self, according to a specific role (lecturer, audience member and so on), much like the space social media platforms occupy, with the front stage being the platform where the user curates and shares content. In the context of this book, this is predominantly health-related, quantifiable self-tracked data or qualitative health-related content (photos of exercising such as yoga mats or landscapes run in, for example).

The 'backstage' 'is a place relative to a given performance, where the impression fostered by the performance is knowingly contradicted as a matter of course' (Goffman, 1959: 112). The backstage, then, is the emotional and intellectual leg work, the how and why users decide to curate and share the many different types of health content that they do, in construction of the 'health self'. This chapter, through presentation of the empirical data that uncovers these backstage deliberations (the interviews and reflexive diary), discusses this navigation for users. In particular, the areas of the backstage are where Hogan argues we do the 'real work', which becomes necessary to 'keep up appearances' (2010: 378). These fronts 'involve the continual adjustment of self-presentation based on the presence of others' (Hogan, 2010: 379). It is also worth mentioning, however, that online we are not always immediately positioned as in front of our audience, and therefore this 'presence of others' is sometimes imagined (as discussed in Chapter 3); thus, the audience or online community (the difference between the two can be acknowledged as contextual) is imagined in the mind of the user, or 'performer'.

Motivations to share

Curating continuity of the digital health self

Sharing self-tracking data or exercise updates provides the participants with a visual documentation and marker to keep themselves accountable to set goals. For example, a participant tracks his daily cycling commute to work as a 'as a marker for myself to aim at as it is the first day back commuting after a break' (Fred, diary entry, 30, M). A desire to post on social media, and to track development after a self-proclaimed 'indulgent' (Christmas) break, ensured that sharing content post-holiday became a significant signpost for letting the social media community know that they were returning to their routine and 'healthy' behaviours. This is demonstrated in Fred's post in Figure 6.1.

This continuity extends to the social media communities' perceptions of the users, and the content is tailored as such. For example, in his final interview, Fred explained that sharing his self-tracking data on social media was for self-surveying purposes, being accountable to himself as well as mitigating potential judgement from his Instagram followers. These fronts 'involve the continual adjustment of self-presentation based on the presence of others' (Hogan, 2010: 379). He does this by explaining it is his 'first ride' back after the Christmas break and also states that this is 'not bad for a chilled ride', alluding to the fact that any break in cycling would explain and justify his slow time and indicating that he was not pushing himself. The following week, Fred provides continuity to this narrative by comparing his time to the status written earlier:

Figure 6.1: Fred's post-Christmas bike ride post

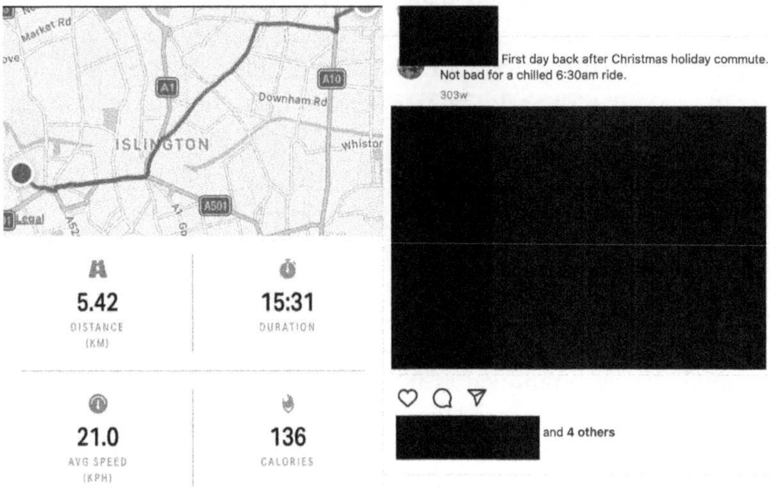
Market Rd
ISLINGTON
Downham Rd
A1
A10
A501
Whiston
5.42
DISTANCE (KM)
15:31
DURATION
21.0
AVG SPEED (KPH)
136
CALORIES
First day back after Christmas holiday commute. Not bad for a chilled 6:30am ride.
303w
and 4 others

> I posted on this day, as it is a week after my first ride back from a winter break. I wanted to see and track whether my performance has improved or worsened (…) I feel the need to follow through in trying to beat my previous post. (Fred, diary entry, 30, M)

By connecting these posts, Fred constructs an online narrative for his social media community. Public diarising of exercise developments speaks to the community through a discourse of self-betterment and improvement, presented in his terms as accountability and competition against himself but also accountability towards an (ever-expanding) online audience. This is examined privately through reflections in his diary:

> Before the start of the ride, I checked on my previous post and was aware of the time and speed to motivate me on this ride. With this in mind I knew where exactly on the journey to push a little bit harder to get a better result. (Fred, diary entry, 30, M)

Therefore, these commuting posts are used by Fred to look back over tracked times and routes, so that he then knows which parts of his journey he needs to improve upon. He could simply use his self-tracking device, without posting, to achieve this, yet sharing provides him with additional evidence and proof of self-improvement. This exploration of the self through data acquisition, which Kristensen and Ruckenstein (2018: 12) conceptualise as a 'laboratory of the self', entails a new awareness of lived experience, where the self is known through data and the data simultaneously informs the self.

As Duffy (2014: np) asserts: 'data scientists are storytellers, interpreters. They take slices of information from the data-sphere around us and translate them into something for us to consume.' However, those constructing the healthy self on social media with their self-tracking become the storytellers. The 'meaning' making from the data visualised extends further than Duffy (2014) proposes here. In fact, rather than providing something for the user to consume (and then share), the visualisations shared on social media are inductive and enable the creation of a data story that 'shape[s] assumptions and promises of visibility and knowing, further connecting to research on how digital devices and the data that they generate configure knowledge spaces in society' (Ruckenstein, 2017: 84). As the continuity of the digital health self, the public narrative provides the social media community with a diary of continual progress through data and self-representations. Therefore, for Fred and for many other users, once this content is shared, the voyeuristic gaze of others serves as a motivating tool for future sharing and exercise practices.

Digital food: moulding bodily consumption to social media aesthetics

For centuries, media representations of food and diet lifestyles have had a huge influence upon cultural meanings associated with what we put in our bodies (Lewis, 2008). As examined in the earlier chapters in this book, whilst data (from self-tracking apps and devices) was often used to represent the body, as a tool to 'share' the body hidden behind the device, it was also used to construct for the eyes of their audience and following an idealised health-conscious and active body, often achieved through content showcasing aesthetically pleasing food and meals. This is often known as 'food porn', 'visual or verbal representations of food that focus intensely on its desire-inducing qualities' (Lupton, 2020: 8). Lifestyle, health and wellness influencers are particularly prone to advocating diet cultures through sharing such content. This becomes particularly problematic and potentially dangerous when circulated by those medically unqualified, as health misinformation is shared to unknowing users who follow such guidance. Whilst this is an alarming and important area of research and also emphasises the need for regulation on social media, it is not the objective of this section, which focuses upon the construction of the health self through digital food sharing by lay users. These users design and mould individual consumption habits to what is aesthetically pleasing to showcase on social media:

> 'I do think when I'm cooking dinner, "ooh this will be a good Instagram picture", so I can think "what can I cook that will look good for Instagram later". I spend so much time moving things around on the plate that by the time I get to eat it it's cold.' (Sophie, first interview, 31, F)

> 'You monitor it. You only show parts of you that you want to show.' (Sophie, first interview, 31, F)

For performers of the 'digital health self', content, in particular food, must be tailored to what is aesthetically pleasing on social media (Kent, 2018, 2020). Satisfaction is felt when food looks 'stylish' (as determined in particular Instagram norms of what is visually pleasing), and thus it is constructed as such (Kent, 2020). For example, they ensured that colourful ingredients were carefully arranged and presented on stylish crockery, conforming to consumer regimes of beauty (Gill, 2007). In contrast, if the meal was not deemed attractive, they felt irritated as they could not share it, especially if they had spent time preparing the meal, and their enjoyment of the food was also diminished because they could not share the image and experience with their social media community. This consideration, therefore, further dictated consumption practices, which prompt users to eat visually and aesthetically pleasing ('healthy') food. These processes of mediation can be analysed through McRobbie's (2009: 62–63) assertion that such 'institutionally unbounded assemblage (…) [produces a] specific subject who is continually dissatisfied about their appearance [or indeed health] and thus compelled to embark on new regimes of "self-perfectibility"'. For example, in her diary, Sophie discussed how she was driven to make meals that she deemed to be 'good' enough for her multiple profiles on Instagram, so she could share them. One example is demonstrated in Figure 6.2.

This self-capitalisation of the visual (Conor, 2004) including the preparation, documentation and sharing of (homemade) meals not only was a labour-intensive process but underlines how users want to have their

Figure 6.2: Sophie's breakfast post

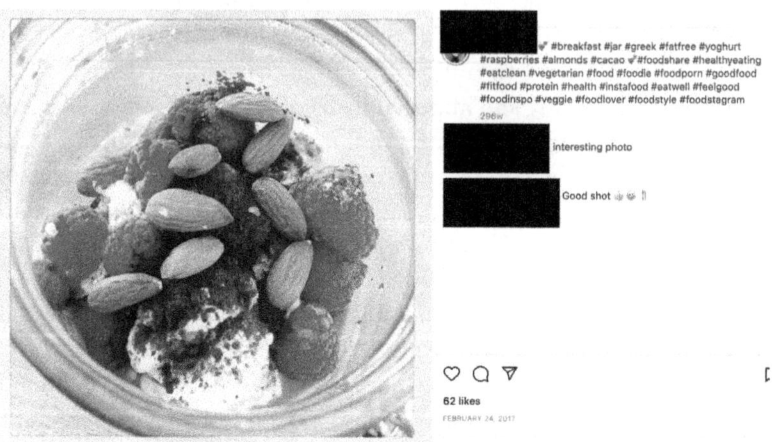

health identity perceived and curated on social media. Time spent shopping for visually pleasing foods as well as their vehicles for presentation (attractive plates, jars and boards) was considered an important and necessary part of the representational and consumption process– from buying the food and crockery, to preparing the meals, to capturing and sharing the image on social media, to finally consuming the meal, reflecting Cederstrom and Spicer's (2015: 7) argument that 'to eat correctly is an achievement, which demonstrates your superior life-skills'. Curating meals that looked attractive and enticing whilst also ensuring their nutritional 'value' contributes to users' own sense of self, of being healthy and productive individuals, whilst also attempting to portray this identity to their social media following. In contrast, users do not always consume foods they enjoy even if nutritionally sound because of their lack of aesthetic value on social media. The 'Insta-worthiness' or 'Insta-grammable' visual aspect of a user's meal or diet dictates what they do and do not consume in daily life.

If we consider this problematic relationship between social media aesthetics, food consumption and digital capitalism, these practices play directly into the hands of the tech giants who commercially profit from the dominant social media companies (in particular, Meta, Tencent and Ali Baba), as well as 'health' and wellness companies and influencers through the exploitation of 'not only the desire to produce an appropriate type of body (with all the symbolism that adheres to it) but also the sense of self-development, mastery, expertise, and skill that dieting [as well as other health or body modifications and representations] can offer' (Heyes, 2006: 137). This 'value' is determined and thus acquired by both the representational 'health' data and the users' sense of feeling 'healthy'. Therefore, the aesthetics of food became integral to not only what these individuals shared online but also what they put in their bodies. Not surprisingly, unattractive representations do not make the final public edit. In turn, the relationship between 'health', lifestyle and diet becomes ever more entwined with these digital food cultures (Lupton, 20202). Exemplified in Figure 6.3 is Lara's post of her after-run 'treat' meal: a 'healthy' wrap from a local deli. This example demonstrates and draws attention to the links between 'healthy' identity construction and the life-stylisation of ethical consumption through self-representations on social media 'symbolising the moral character and identity of the user' (Baker and Walsh, 2020: 54):

As Lara asserted:

> I shared a photo of my after-run treat – a wrap from a local deli – which serves super healthy fast food. I love the food there and it was part of my motivation as I was running – I was chanting the name of the deli as it was going to keep me going. I knew I was going to share a pic of it as I was running – I thought it would be a different thing

Figure 6.3: Lara's post-run treat meal

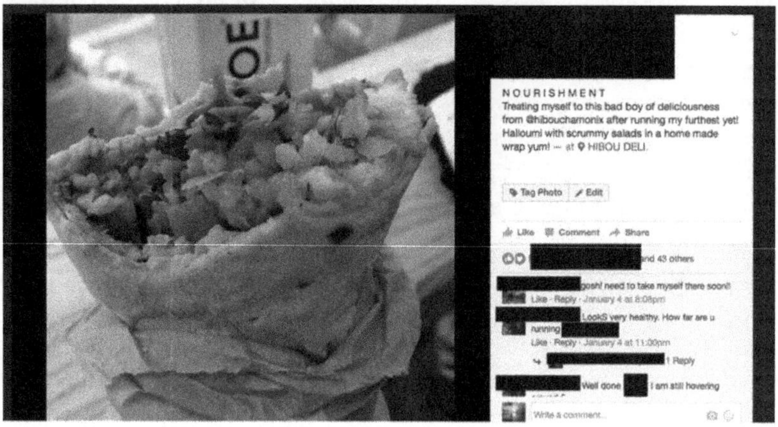
NOURISHMENT
Treating myself to this bad boy of deliciousness from @hibouchamonix after running my furthest yet! Halloumi with scrummy salads in a home made wrap yum! — at HIBOU DELI.
Tag Photo
Edit
Like
Comment
Share
and 43 others
gosh! need to take myself there soon!!
Like · Reply
LookS very healthy. How far are u running
Like · Reply
1 Reply
Well done
I am still hovering
Write a comment...

> to post regarding my running logs on Instagram. I also like promoting local businesses and would recommend this particular place to anyone visiting Chamonix. (Lara, diary entry, 28, F)

This quote from Lara's reflexive diary explains how 'delicious' and healthy food became a mantra to motivate further running as well as sharing the image with her social media community to provide a 'variety' of ethical and healthy content. This discourse illustrates the argumentation I set out in Chapter 4 and elsewhere (Kent, 2018, 2020, 2021), where I discuss how food and morality have an established history and how moral values become ascribed to 'good' or 'bad' foods. For users posting 'healthy treat meals' (whether consciously or not), in turn postulates that eating 'bad' foods is associated with some moral inferiority and 'good' healthy foods contribute to some kind of moral superiority (Baker and Walsh, 2020). Exercising is considered a healthy goal so as to be rewarded by eating a favourite 'healthy' food afterwards, but for the digital health self, the reward is also to share this content for diversity of representation as well as performance of the moral character of the individual.

Life-stylisation of the digital health self

The different types of content and self-representations shared on social media by users ideologically and discursively conveyed different health identities and determinants in the performance of what is 'healthy' for the online community. As Mennel et al (1992: 36) explain: 'the social value attached to food, health and physical beauty has risen constantly in the second half of the twentieth century', thus blurring the ideological boundaries between 'health' and 'lifestyle' (Lewis, 2008; Cederstrom and Spicer, 2015; Davies, 2016; Moore 2017). This has only been further exacerbated as performing health and lifestyle practices become a normalised daily habit for users of social media and those self-tracking their health. This section will examine in depth the representational tools participants employed to enable such life-stylisation of the digital health self and why this became such an effective discourse in their 'healthy' identity creation. For many users styling representations of 'healthy' behaviours and exercise in locations they visited was a common practice. Enjoyment of the beautiful surroundings was 'enhanced' by exercising in these locations as well as providing a scenic backdrop for social media content sharing, and receiving positive feedback from the online community, relating to both exercising and the picturesque setting, also provided additional pleasure. As Lou described:

> 'Distance I think is something that is interesting to share because actually the first question I'd always get was "oh my god how far did you run this weekend?" I'd say "16 miles" and they'd say, "that's so ridiculous". In terms of stats, speed and hills climbed, I find it a quite self-indulgent thing to share. It's almost too much bragging. For me, my sharing was kind of influenced by the fact that I wasn't necessarily staying out as late as other people, because I needed to go home because I needed to get up the next day. I wasn't going to all the events I should have been going to or I'd be arriving late to it because I had to do a run in the morning. I think for me it was a bit more of that social side of sharing, being like "I am still doing cool stuff, I am still going to cool places."' (Lou, final interview, 29, F)

Simply sharing screenshots of self-tracked distances (for the runners) from apps was often considered uninteresting by the sharers themselves. Therefore, users life-styled their posts (as we see from Figures 6.4 and 6.5) by taking pictures of where they were going, often in attempt make their lifestyle more relatable to others. Exercising in a beautiful location for one's own enjoyment was not always or often the motivation here, as demonstrated later in this chapter. Sometimes this desire to capture a 'picturesque' running location or an aesthetically pleasing meal, detracted from the participants' enjoyment of what they were actually doing, the exercise or eating. In this way, health becomes, to an extent, collaborative as users exercise in aesthetically pleasing locations to document this and share for the attention of their social media community. These practices extend Lucivero and Prainsack's (2015) arguments that self-tracking technologies are lifestyle products, which in today's digital society blur the boundaries between regulated medical devices and consumer products. Not only does capturing 'health' become life-stylised with these ambiguously defined

Figure 6.4: Lou's woodland image life-stylisation of health

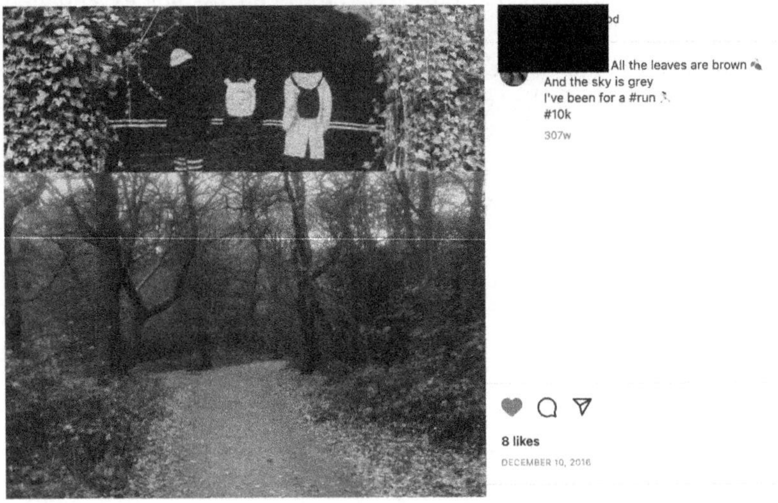
All the leaves are brown
And the sky is grey
I've been for a #run
#10k
307w
8 likes
DECEMBER 10, 2016

Figure 6.5: Examples of participant-shared content – life-stylisation of health (cycling)

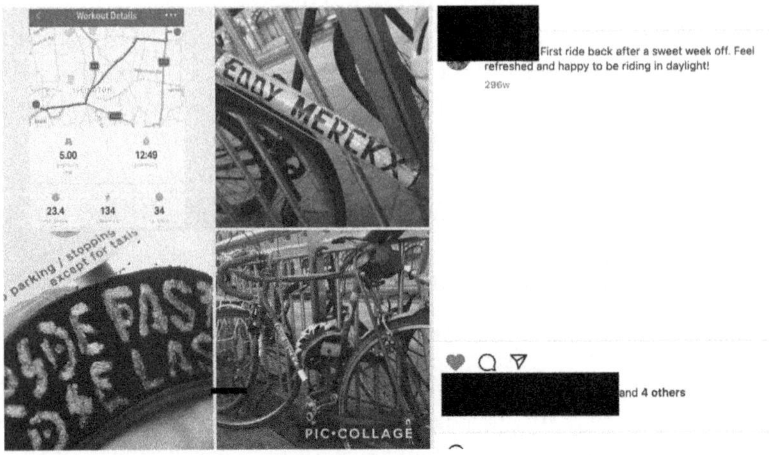
Workout Details
5.00
12:49
23.4
134
34
parking / stopping except for taxis
PIC·COLLAGE
First ride back after a sweet week off. Feel refreshed and happy to be riding in daylight!
296w
and 4 others

and (not always regulated) devices, but so too do exercise and evidence of 'health' through representations on social media. 'Healthy' behaviours are enacted by the individual, captured and represented on social media for their own benefits as well as for the community, who through feedback loops on social media platforms simultaneously become a part of the health identity of the sharer online and offline. This is 'reconstituting the norms of living and living as a human subject' (Clough, 2010: 11), through the use of technologies of the self. These processes affect and in turn encourage the participants, either through pressurising influences or pleasurable motivations for 'healthy' offline behaviours. These life-stylisations of 'health' also became a form of public diarising for the participants in the sense that they felt it represented some of their identity, not just their health. As Sophie asserts:

> 'I guess it's almost like a diary for yourself, a public diary even though you're not going to be as honest in a diary online that is public and online about something that is private.' (Sophie, final interview, 31, F)

Sharing 'health' practices on social media, therefore, can be used as a form of logging public life and memory, to look back over 'health' developments but also all aspects of the participants' lifestyles. Walker-Rettberg understands such digital self-presentation as 'cumulative, rather than presented as a physical whole' (2015: 5); through a collection of posts and micro narratives users contribute to a curated image, showing not all but some of their public life. These carefully curated and mediated representations take a huge amount of the participants' time and require technological literacy to achieve the desired effects. In this regard, the life-stylisation of 'health' includes the documentation of fitness and skill progression, as well as technological fluency. Lifestyle becomes ever more entwined with body image and identity when being represented through the digital health self in these data-sharing cultures.

Social media etiquettes

Gendered, idealised and sexualised bodies

Instagram, in contrast to Facebook, was seen as the most appropriate platform by users wanting to share specific sexualised photos of their bodies. Facebook was used to upload more images and write in more narrative forms about daily lifestyle and health goals (met). Instagram, perhaps unsurprisingly, was more focused on the visual documentation and representation of health, with a 'less is more' approach, less quantity but a better perceived quality of images. These findings support a wealth of literature that argues how social media, in particular Instagram, greatly impacts self-construction of gender (Blower, 2016). This leads to damaging sexualisation and problematic objectification of both male and female bodies and how 'the role of sexuality in these online environments holds major influence in this self-construction' (Davis, 2018: 1). These are unregulated and potentially toxic environments for many but particularly young users when it comes to body image (Garcia-Gomez, 2017, *Wall Street Journal*, 15 September 2021) and the negative impacts made on users' self-esteem and mental health when comparisons to other users' lifestyles are made (Kent, 2020a, 2020b).

> Instagram was basically stills' of the same – fitness selfie, food and the gym. I'm using Instagram for a sexier approach as this seems to reel in all the fitness fanatics so photos, I post on here would not usually go on other platforms. I also posted a booty progress update – as I am doing this weekly at the moment. (Annie, diary entry, 28, F)

In the context of health performativity, users frequently adhered to the discourse of 'health' being 'sexy' and desirable. To gain more followers, users sexualised their content, showing more skin, and slim, toned figures, and posed in provocative ways for gym selfies, for example; this was the representational strategy to gain more 'followers' and exposure on Instagram. This resonates with Heyes' (2006: 137) assertion: 'The social rewards that accrue to being slim are very real.' Heyes attributes the cycle of dieting, of 'elation' and 'failure', to a sense of reincarnation through self-organisation. The 'hyperbolic construction of "success stories"' (Heyes, 2006: 145) contribute to this inequality as the narrated fabrications denote a discourse of reincarnation of one's self and body, which is potentially achievable or always just out of reach. These findings demonstrate the rise of aesthetic self-tracking (Elias et al, 2017) and the normalisation of positioning (representations of) our bodies as subjects of excellence (Gill and Scharff, 2011). These 'entrepreneurial modes of selfhood [are] centred on labour, measurement, comparison and (self-)transformation' (Elias and Gill, 2017: 3) and increasing pervasive surveillance of the self and others. Lara reflected on this in her diary entry:

> When I look at Instagram, it is mainly at photography and yoga accounts. I do think I want to look a certain way and doing exercise regularly is a way of achieving that, I'm now trying to do that. (Lara, diary entry, 28, F)

However, these representations of, particularly female, bodies conformed to slim, sexualised and idealised body shapes, and because of this, the other participants felt that if they could not conform to these same bodily ideals with their images, they had to consider what they could 'get away with' posting. What must be recognised here is that in my research study only half the research participants were female. None of the male participants mentioned any concern about wanting or avoiding sexual or thin-ideal objectification of their bodies. Overall, these findings extend Rettberg's (2014) important argument that asserts that technological filters are entangled with cultural ones. Beauty apps do much more than simply reinforcing established cultural ideas about (female) attractiveness. They contribute to the '"anestheticising" and "(de)familisaring" effect of seeing ourselves through technological–cultural filters' (Rettberg, 2014: 25–26). Worryingly, not feeling attractive 'enough' to be sharing images of their bodies for fear of negative judgement from others online was a real concern and pressure for most of the female users. None of the male users highlighted this as a personal concern at this stage of the research study. As Lara stated:

> I shared a selfie of my run onto Instagram and Facebook; I nearly didn't add it onto Facebook as I don't really like the photo (…) I was more focused on the run than taking a 'nice' picture, but it was all I had so went for it. I feel there are a larger group of people on Facebook to see and judge I guess, but I was pleasantly surprised that people were really supportive, and it gave me a boost. I want to keep at it – the running I mean, not posting selfies! (Lara, diary entry, 28, F)

Overall, interestingly, Facebook was perceived to be more 'public' than Instagram as (both male and female) users had more 'friends' on the platform, which enabled a broader context collapse of networks, for example, links with friends, family, acquaintances and colleagues past, present and potentially future. Instagram, therefore, was perceived as less judgemental, as participants tended not to have 'followers' and networks linked with all aspects of their lives. They, therefore, felt that this was less worrying in terms of what content they shared and how they may be perceived, especially for those users training towards specific goals. As Annie reflected:

> 'I plan on just taking a backseat and building myself up, I'll do a lot more on Instagram definitely. I'll be swapping over platforms a bit I think, less pressure on Instagram.' (Annie, final interview, 28, F)

Therefore, the perceived judgement imagined through Facebook was diminished when sharing on Instagram. Instagram was conceived as a safer and more private space, enabling the sharing of imperfect pictures, personal information or storytelling. These findings support Trottier's (2012) work on interpersonal surveillance and Moore's (2017) work on self-tracking in the workplace, which both identify how users' perceptions and management of their own visibility online and the visibility of others are tied to shifting understandings of what is considered public and private information. Lara reflected on this in her final interview:

> 'I feel like Facebook is a lot more public, I feel like Instagram is a lot more journal-ly, (…) so maybe that's a side that supports mental health. I don't know. I still feel that mental health has a bit of a stigma the way

> people view it as "oversharing". Someone's commented on one of my photos and I then went onto hers and there is a lot of disturbing stuff out there. She was into suicide survival. It was all very depressing on her page and it was all very vocal about stuff that a lot of people do keep personal, but I was wondering how encouraging that was and if that was healthy or not.' (Lara, final interview, 28, F)

Instagram was perceived by all the participants as a platform for journaling or diarising. Due to the stigmas attached to mental health issues and eating disorders, Instagram was, compared to Facebook and other social media platforms (Twitter, Snapchat and so on), perceived as more private and therefore supportive to tackle, document or discuss personal (mental health) issues. Annie interestingly reframed this in a utopian way and articulated her use of Instagram like a 'goal board':

> 'It's like scrolling through my own desires, my own wants, I use it to inspire me to better myself rather than caring about what anyone else is up to right now.' (Annie, final interview, 28, F)

In this way, Instagram enabled the participants to conceptualise their individual desires, wants and ambitions and this data to be subsequently visualised and 'liked', captured and documented, and returned to as a companion (Rettberg, 2018). However, as Talbot et al (2017) identified, the repetition of images of the body ideal, which is an often unattainable and unrealistic construction of both feminine beauty and masculine strength, can lead to a decrease in body satisfaction. Although Talbot et al (2017) were researching 'thinspiration', 'fitspiration' and 'bonespiration' images shared on social media, and this analysis does not focuses on the circulation of thin-ideal shared content, there are overlaps between 'thinspiration' and 'health-related content' in terms of their damaging impact upon both the female sharers and their audiences as regards how they perceive and judge their bodies. More worryingly perhaps, content that prompted healthy practices and 'fitspiration' was often perceived by sharers and their communities as 'allegedly healthy' and 'mentally better' than 'thinspiration' content. Yet it contained very similar imagery of particularly female bodies: thin and toned. Problematically, recent research by the Mental Health Foundation (2020 Body Image Report) identified that 20 per cent of adults and 40 per cent of teenagers say images on social media cause them to worry about their body image. Although the participants attempted not to conform to the visually idealised body image and shapes, this was often impossible in these comparative data-sharing health communities. As Talbot et al (2017: 5) explained, the 'everyday user could, therefore, be at risk of viewing this potentially harmful content that idealises the extremely thin female body'. Although the participants used Facebook and Instagram to share different content in different ways, this was often with a preconception of how those imagined communities would perceive and potentially judge it (Anderson, 1983). Instagram provided participants with a space for more personal diarising, and Facebook enabled broader and higher quantities of content to be shared. Yet both afforded the participants a platform to represent idealised 'healthy' bodies and identities, or at least notions of what that could and they hoped to look like.

Balancing oversharing and showing off

Within these sharing communities there is a 'trade off' between managing privacy and achieving public exposure (Tufecki, 2008; Boyd and Hargittai, 2010). Mediated representations of the self are often carefully constructed to demonstrate 'authenticity' of content and character in an attempt to not 'overshare'. Personal branding online becomes synonymous with authenticity, without perhaps a recognition that authenticity is very much a social construct (Sternberg, 1998). Broadly, 'oversharing' refers to both the frequency of posts as well as the content determined as inauthentic or desiring of attention (Kent, 2018: 66–67). Oversharing is associated with attention-seeking gratification, which is negatively perceived by others within the community. If self-censorship is not appropriately maintained, sharing of certain health practices is perceived (whether real or imagined) by the wider community in a critical light as 'oversharing' (Kent, 2018: 67). Using social media platforms to celebrate individual achievements or goals met was a key motivator to share content online. 'Showing off' in this manner, however, was interestingly achieved in different ways and for many different reasons. As discussed earlier in this chapter, Lara life-stylised many of her marathon training posts:

> 'If I was out on a run and I happened to see something that looked nice, I might take a picture and then casually drop in that that was on a run. You still are then hinting to people, "I go running."' (Lara, final interview, 28, F)

Rather than explicitly stating training goals, she shared posts of places she visited to 'hint' that she was running. She explained that this felt less attention-seeking. For Tim, 'showing off' was framed through feelings of pride:

> My post contained a video of myself doing yoga (as most do!) It was something I'd been practicing for a while, I wanted to share it a little bit out of pride for my hard work and progress. (Tim, diary entry, 34, M)

'Showing off' health and fitness progress provided additional gratification for the participants but interestingly did not prevent them from continuing to share similar content. As Roy attested:

> It's a way to share things with my friends. It took me a while to get over the hurdle of being viewed as a show-off (which is very prominent in my offline social circle), but if sharing the things I do interests other people, why not? (Roy, diary entry, 26, M)

Roy acknowledges that some of his sharing practices were considered attention-seeking from his offline social circle. Yet this legitimated his sharing because he considered the community and voyeurs online as wanting to see his updates. This resonated with Goffman's (1959: 139) arguments that the balance between sharing (performing) and concealing is mediated by the traditions of a group or social status. Furthermore, showing off was also practiced and mitigated by the frequency of the participants' posts. Unspoken yet clear community etiquettes in these data-sharing cultures outlined that regular posting was expected (as examined in Chapter 5). Yet regular 'showing off' was deemed to be 'oversharing' within these communities. Therefore, posting regularly but not *too regularly* was key. As Roy stated:

> 'It's something that annoys me in other people, like when someone has six videos in a row. It's like "I like seeing your stuff and I like talking with you", but I do not need to see every single bit of your workout.' (Roy, final interview, 26, M)

Therefore, quantity over quality of content was deemed oversharing. In Roy and many of the participants' terms this was exemplified by showing 'every' bit of your workout, rather than one image. This was considered too much information (colloquially, TMI). Continual adjustments, therefore, were made regarding what and how much content was posted and performed, in relation to the (perceived) judgement from the community (Marwick and boyd, 2010). Oversaturation of content was considered by the participants to devalue it in some intangible way. Interestingly, Roy provided a comparable offline example of this:

> 'It's like when you meet someone on the street and you start talking about something and maybe they tell you about what they do. Oversharing is like also telling you where they live, how their childhood was, if their Mum or Dad was around. It's like "I don't need this stuff – why are you sharing this for."' (Roy, final interview, 26, M)

To overshare then was conceived as stemming from the (over)sharer lacking something in their personal life, a type of 'wanting' and a need to fulfil a personal emotional void (Gilroy-Ware, 2017). The same could be said of oversharing in the offline world, that the sharers required when needing emotional support, help or advice. As Sophie expanded:

> 'My motivation I guess for sharing was to get acknowledgement from people that I'm doing well and feel good about myself. There is a definitely an element of wanting to show off too, definitely the habitual thing of just wanting (...) gratification, generally people want to be loved. They want people to like them, they want to feel good about themselves. It's quite a selfish thing, because people generally don't post because they think I genuinely want to help someone today. You post because you want to feel good about yourself.' (Sophie, final interview, 31, F)

Most of the participants were concerned about being perceived as show-offs and being judged poorly by their communities. For Tim, there was a tension between wanting to post and update his community, gaining attention and not wanting to 'show off':

> 'I do get mixed feelings on posting and the amount of people that might see or comment on that. I guess just from a point of view that I want to post things, to share what I'm doing, to share my happiness and pride in what I've achieve and progressed in and if that can inspire a few people, then that's cool, I really like that. If I get a little private message saying "oh, Tim, I'm really loving this and I'm going to give it a try" or "it's put a smile on my face today", I love that because that's really nice. But then if it's a load of people saying it then I feel a bit, not insecure, that maybe it's gone to another place that I don't necessarily want.' (Tim, final interview, 34, M)

Here we see some interesting tensions between sharing content being seen as 'showing off' and a simultaneous feeling of gratification gained through feedback and the 'likes' on these types of posts. The participants experienced an internal conflict between appearing (as well as personally feeling) too desiring of attention and wanting to share. Tim referenced this when he stated that 'I wouldn't want to have a post that would have you know hundreds of likes and loads of people saying you're great, "this inspired me". I'd really struggle with that' (Tim, final interview, 34, M).

A certain amount of 'likes' or feedback can make the user feel exposed or attention-seeking. Roy, in the final interview, when reflecting upon his diary entries and social media posting more generally, expressed contradictory traits. He expressed emphatically that he did not like being the object of the community's gaze and did not identify as enjoying being the centre of attention. Yet sometimes he automatically shared things as a 'no brainer', which legitimated it as being in the community's interest.

As briefly discussed in the previous section, sharing to fulfil a need that perhaps was not being met in the participant's personal life was a motivator to share and 'show off' on social media. This was identified as becoming a habit, a sense of feeling good about oneself because the community 'liked' the participant's lifestyle, personal activities or events, as evidenced in their posts. This was recognised as additionally gratifying when the participant had not posted for some time due to personal events. As Annie wrote, '[I] posted a couple of photos about Matt and I signing out tenancy today (…) It felt nice to have something to post about!! I felt happy to share our happiness with the world' (Annie, diary entry, 28, F).

In addition, sharing any life event unrelated to health, for example, ensured the participants' 'happiness' was considered legitimate to 'show off' and share with the wider community, particularly when they had not for personal reasons been able to post for some time. The participants experienced frustration at not being able to post and felt a desire and compulsion to contribute regularly to their online narrative and idealised 'healthy' self and lifestyle.

Conclusions

Capturing and sharing health and lifestyle on social media have become an outlet and medium for autobiographical narratives, personal storytelling and self-tracking and a form of public diarising for users. Balancing content and mediations between platforms (for my participants this was, in particular, Facebook and Instagram) to construct desired healthy identities in consideration of each platform's own socio-technological affordances and community etiquettes, performing the digital health self can be situated within the sharing of health-related content and a variety of representations of an 'idealised' active body in social media spaces. Users become subjected to the normalised gaze of what is performed as 'healthy' online (as illustrated in Chapter 1), as well as their own self-surveillance of who to become. Those sharing flawless portraits of personal identity by showing off representative and desirable personality traits to peers and anonymous evaluators (van Dijck, 2013b: 208). The digital health self can be a construction of a health identity that other users within the social media community could perceive and connect with, an often-utopian idealised representation of a healthy user. These constructions are carefully edited to show the achievements and goals met, idealised visual representations of the body and the life-stylisation of consumption habits, which reinforce self-betterment discourses of the 'healthy' subject (Fotopoulou and O'Riordan, 2016).

Although this chapter presented and examined qualitative representations of 'health' more than data from self-tracking devices for instance, habitually sharing these self-representations of health-related behaviours contributes to a form of lifelogging of 'health', which we can also identify in the construction of a 'health' identity through quantitative data. Furthermore, as Gilmore (2015: 2532) argues, quantitative data transforms personal experience and 'is apt to provoke a qualitative transformation of experience predicated on the technology's social aspects. The quantified self, in other words, actually promotes a qualitative re-experience of our bodies and our social relationships.' The social relationships forged online (built from both online and offline networks) by the participants centred around representations of specific identities, in this case as 'healthy' and transforming individuals. The accumulation of shared content related and necessary to perform 'healthy' identities forms a quantitative logging, categorisation and classification of the self, whereby the body is represented and moulded to conform to the desired aesthetics of social media. Therefore, within data-sharing 'health' cultures, digital technologies provoke the online body and the offline self to frequently meet in a troublesome dialect whereby diet and the body are tailored and sculpted to the preferred aesthetics of what is visually pleasing on social media, rather than what these individuals may personally desire to eat or to do for exercise. The digital health self, then, prioritises performativity of the body and its consumption or exercise needs, sometimes over their relationship with personal preferences. Does preference of food or exercise shift towards those that *are* easily captured and demonstrate the curated healthy self? Is it arguable then that over time this body might consistently desire behaviours or foods that can be framed and captured in digestible and engaging social media worthy content?

7

Future Directions for the Digital Health Self

This book provides a unique contribution to the expanding literature on self-tracking technologies and social media through its analysis of users' practices of using these technologies to self-represent 'health' identities and how such performances under the online communities' gaze affected their 'health' behaviours and practices offline. Much research has now attended to the use of self-tracking technologies in multiple settings such as work and insurance schemes, schools, leisure pursuits and in self-tracking communities (Lupton, 2014, 2016a; Fotopoulou and O'Riordan, 2016; Ajana, 2017; Goodyear et al, 2017; Moore, 2017; Kristensen and Prigge, 2018; Moore et al, 2018; Rettberg, 2018; Ruffino, 2018;Spiller et al, 2018; Till, 2018). However, this research has addressed a gap in the literature, which so far has failed to examine the user perspective in the use of these technologies to perform health on social media and how these curated 'health' identities affect users' 'health' behaviours in their everyday 'offline' lives. Neoliberal rationalities, which have 'fundamental preference for the market over the state as a means of resolving problems and achieving human ends' (Crouch, 2011: 7), have shifted public and digital health practices towards self-care through discourses of self-responsibilisation. Self-tracking technologies have largely evaded critique and have primarily been promoted as revolutionary tools for health betterment; they assist with reflexive management of individual risk (Nettleton and Burrows, 2003; Moore and Robinson, 2016) and assume that the accumulation of 'health' information and the 'datafication of health' (Ruckenstein and Schull, 2017: 262) are better for individual wellbeing. This is a product of wide corporate systemic structures and neoliberal free market strategies of individualised health practices and self-management, adopted by citizens in their construction of identities, for themselves and their communities, to be responsible 'healthy' and morally 'good' citizens. Within these neoliberal frames, the body becomes subordinated through adoption of technology and control of the mind (Moore and Robinson, 2016).

Broadly speaking, these technologies challenge and shape understandings of how we interpret our everyday environment and health knowledge. Individual 'health' has become collaborative in these data-sharing spheres; as mentioned in Chapter 6, 'healthy' behaviours are enacted by the individual, captured and represented on social media for their own benefits as well as for the community, who through feedback loops simultaneously become a part of the 'health' identity of the sharer online. In turn, this affects and encourages 'healthy' online behaviours, either through peer pressure or pleasurable motivation. Thus, we have to ask, are these pressures or motivations ever mentally 'healthy' for individual wellbeing? This question is particularly pertinent when we consider that the line between stress, pleasure and motivation becomes ever more interlocked in these social media and data-sharing communities. This concluding chapter will present a summary and discussion of the empirical research findings presented throughout this book, of the everyday impact of self-tracking and social media upon mental and physical health.

Self and community surveillance in digital health practices

Self-surveillance through self-monitoring has been viewed as 'empowering' (Beato, 2012), enabling users to take control of their 'health' and body, externally from health institutions and wider surveillance, making 'behaviour change easy, inexpensive, and unobtrusive' (Swan, 2012b: 112). This book has interrogated claims about the technological health revolution promised by digital health technologies by exploring the influence and impact of self-tracking health technologies upon individual health behaviours and constructions of the self. There is some literature recognising the persuasive and at times coercive design of self-tracking technologies (Purpura et al, 2011). However, this book carried out a detailed analysis focusing upon the regulatory design of digital health technologies and impacts upon decision making around 'health' practices. 'Empowerment' was temporal, and relatively short-lived, as most participants who adopted self-tracking tools did so to achieve personal targets (doing marathons or reaching weight-lifting goals, for example). Because of the continual monitoring and sharing of these practices via these technologies and social media, self-regulation and self-discipline did become overwhelming, forcing participants to 'digitally detox' (take a break from social media for weeks/months) or quit altogether. Furthermore, the continual comparisons and competitions of life(style) representation on social media highlighted individuals' voids or perceived 'inadequacies' in their own lives and in their own bodies.

In many cases, sharing content deemed 'personal' or 'transparent' caused embarrassment when considering the gaze of the community. Self-censorship, therefore, is actively managed, based upon perceived negative judgement from community members. Self-surveillance through peer surveillance, then, becomes an individualised pressure for users. This, in turn, may encourage a detachment from the community and the observed nature of sharing 'health' informatics to avoid additional pressures felt from the gaze of others. The representation of 'healthy' identities is achieved through, for and with the help of the audience. Surveillance of and by others influences self-tracking users' practices of self-presentation. The information produced through these devices changes users' behaviours and understandings of their bodies and what is deemed as 'healthy', which are reinforced by the feedback received from the social media community. Users tended to feel 'healthier' through sharing 'health'-related data on social media.

These digital and data-sharing cultures provide ways of experiencing and viewing one's own body and 'health' in relation to others, meaning health-related behaviours have become intimately linked to constructions of the idealised digital health self enabled through social media performativity. The representations of this identity online and self-tracking health behaviours offline form an interdependent process. The value of surveillance in this regard plays a dominant role in these data-sharing cultures. Self-tracking means that 'health' is now managed and controlled through technological devices, reducing human health and senses to those decipherable only through computer senses, which are calculable, efficient and predictable (Ritzer et al, 2012), as well as profitable and commercially mined. In these research findings good 'health' was equated to being fit and most importantly doing exercise (regardless of how frequently or how much was in reality achieved). Not being 'fat' or overweight was another signifier of being 'healthy' (Powell and Fitzpatrick, 2015). In this regard, users 'quantified' 'health' numerically by counting calories consumed or by having parameters for what they determined was a personal 'healthy' weight, regardless of other lifestyle behaviours (poor food consumption or lack of exercise, for example). Sense of self was not considered something permanent; 'health' identities were considered as something that could be transformed, through self-surveillance and self-tracking the body, thus overcoming its perceived limitations.

Social media functions as a social venue to represent health practices. The digital health self-presentation is carefully constructed under the consciousness of peer surveillance and (imagined) observation of others within social media. These constructions are arguably possible only for a highly reflexive individual (Giddens, 1991) who is continually involved in self-monitoring, both online and offline. Subscribing to discourses of 'self-betterment' using self-tracking, in whatever capacity that was individually determined, meant that the embodiment of 'good health' and feeling morally 'better' and physically 'well' was enabled and supported through the accountability of sharing data and progress with participatory audiences. Most interestingly, receiving feedback and being under the gaze of social media communities (both public and private networks) make users feel well and healthy regardless of their actual developments or improvements; if their community deemed them 'healthy', self-trackers embodied the community's gaze of health admiration.

Self-presentation online is carefully constructed through a balance between exposure and concealment of offline behaviours and specific 'health' practices. Sharing self-tracking practices is also intended for surveillance by the community on social media (real or imagined). The gaze of the others increases the pressure on the user to respond to and in turn represent their digital health practice through certain 'healthy' signs. 'Health', therefore, is identified as being intertwined with many different areas of one's lifestyle, meaning the sharing of self-tracking practices on social media becomes integral to the users' everyday habits and to the wider online community, in terms of contributing to their sense of self as 'healthy' or 'unhealthy' individuals. Perceived relevance is key when these individuals decide between what to post and where, which was informed by platform-specific social media etiquettes. Pervasive tracking, sharing and surveillant practices dominate these users' daily lives, with their online and offline realms inseparable; for these individuals, there is no divide, nor is it distinct, and so, the wall between them is increasingly porous and fluid.

Committing to health 'optimisation' via social media sharing

Within this book representations of the body, and of 'healthy' identities came both from social media and self-tracking technologies. Both the process of capturing and sharing qualitative representations of 'health' (fitness or gym selfies or 'food photography', for example) and more quantitative representations of 'health' (self-tracking data, for example), for self- and peer surveillance and self-motivations, enabled 'healthier' activities for 'self-betterment' and 'self optimisation'. These user cultures and practices of 'health' management and improvement were situated within market economy discourses, and through self-tracking technologies and social media affordances, their self-representations could be neatly packaged, branded and commodified within the capitalist cycle of consumerism. 'Health', then, became recognised within a discourse of commodification: a numerical or captured packaging of the self through representational data and a product that could be easily shared and circulated between communities, not always considering that this was sold (to third parties) for data mining. Through these practices, the users were able to instruct, regulate, normalise and represent a curated and idealised notion of the active 'healthy' subject: the digital health self. These standards of judgement were conformed to through 'consumer welfare', which 'is needed [to determine] against which competitive behaviour is to be criticised and periodically stopped' (Davies, 2015: 63). Such 'consumer welfare' consists of the adoption of self-tracking technologies and devices and subsequent representations on social media to consume and perform competitive and comparative 'healthy' lifestyles that comply with these neoliberal standards and their implied judgements. The continual representational practices that were embraced adhered to a commodification of the self (Ursell, 2000), through individualising and sharing practices. Their perceptions and representations of self and 'health' management reflected very clearly neoliberal self-responsibilisation (Crouch, 2011; Cederstrom and Spicer, 2015; Davies, 2015, 2016). Forlano (2013: 2) argues that this real and virtual hybrid space speaks to 'a need for notions of place that specify the ways in which people, place, and technology are interdependent, relational and mutually constituted'. This book, therefore, has attended to the use of self-tracking technologies and social media's performative capacities whilst recognising that we do not make choices to construct our 'health' identities in a social, cultural or economic vacuum. Thus, the online community serves as a mediatory sphere from which to affect behaviours through feedback or a lack thereof, as much as providing the technological tools that can guide users' behaviours under digital capitalism's desire for data sharing and the monetisation of our attention.

By sharing health and fitness-related posts, self-trackers became representative of a community of like-minded 'health'-orientated individuals, which they – even when nothing was being personally achieved – felt part of. This positively and optimistically contributed to their sense of self and identity as informed, educated and improving 'healthy' beings. However, when they experienced stress or trauma in their personal lives, the concealment of 'unhealthy' behaviours to avoid the negative judgement of others relieved them from being the object of the communities' gaze and judging their own lives through comparing lifestyles represented and surveilled on social media. Interestingly, what good 'health' meant was subjectively interpreted by all the participants in this research, but surprisingly, they all exhibited a commitment to 'health' in whatever goal-orientated capacity that was individually determined. Commitments to 'health', being 'healthier' and 'getting fitter' (through exercise and consumption practices), became the focal point in dictating and controlling lifestyle and 'health'-related behaviours. Commitments to being 'healthy' were so subjectively interpreted that being 'healthy' at times almost lost its meaning and became muddied by over-regulatory commitments to self-tracking and 'personal rehabilitation' (Cederstrom and Spicer, 2015: 134). Self-trackers' processes of 'committing' to health goals over time became the dominant guide, embodying a commitment to regulation and self-optimisation, regardless of any impacts upon physical health or mental wellbeing. Interestingly, the regulatory use of these technologies was extremely influential over health behaviours, advocating a moralism of 'health' internalised through privatised self-policing but which over time detrimentally affected their sense of self-worth and wellbeing.

Restrictive notions of 'healthiness'

These technologies challenge and shape our social values, meanings and understandings of how we interpret our bodies. When the body is reduced to data and then represented through self-tracking devices and social media, an oversimplification of the body and 'health' occurs. This has implications for how bodies function and operate in terms of parameters of 'good' or 'bad', 'healthy' or 'unhealthy', individuals and lifestyles. Conceiving the interplay between, relationship with and construction of these technologies as a means of representing the body, the biological and health, this book has challenged the limiting concept of the 'data double', which is a reductionist representation of the monitored body (Whitson and Haggerty, 2008: 574). The 'meaning' making from the data visualised extends further than has been proposed (Duffy, 2014).

Creating personal and social media narratives from our quantified data helps make our self-tracking data relatable, personal and humanised. In fact, rather than providing something for the user to consume (and then share if they so wish), the visualisations are inductive and a creation of a data story. As de Certeau's (1984: 129) asserts: 'what the map cuts up, the story cuts across.' A positive perspective would view this online trail as an individual story. A negative perspective would consider it as conducive to control and surveillance. The negative impacts on 'health' and wellbeing resulting from using these technologies stemmed mostly from the dominating, regulatory and self-disciplining behaviours the participants adopted. These behaviours may to an extent empower an individual in optimising their 'health'. However, in a neoliberal age, where individualising self-regulatory practices are discursively advocated through the distancing of state support, individuals are reduced to consumers, and personal 'health' is now a commodity to be packaged and shared. This book, therefore, does not consider the state as 'a force with necessarily clean hands' (Crouch, 2011: 172). The promotion and practice of self-tracking can then be readily conceived as an embodiment of the neoliberal individualised practices the state and corporations of late consumer capitalism have enforced upon its citizens (Moore and Robinson, 2016; Moore, 2017).

Much of the literature around self-tracking discusses the positives that can be drawn from an abundance of data. In this research study, self-achievement was experienced through the self-evidence of data, which to an extent meant that the acquisition of data enabled individuals to feel 'healthier'. Personal discovery and revelation were often enabled through these self-surveying practices and data acquisitions. The participants found them conducive to tell 'more' about their bodies, and 'health' was identified as becoming intricately entwined with their sense of self, as 'good' or 'bad', 'healthy' or 'unhealthy', individuals. They used this data and self-representations online to 'make sense of the world around them' (Duffy, 2014: np). In turn, the distinctions between the physical body, data and the mind were renegotiated and shifted their normative definitions and understandings of what they considered a 'body', a person (Datteri and Tamburrini, 2009), 'health' and lifestyle. In turn, this shifted definitions of what they deemed 'healthy' or 'unhealthy' individuals and bodies, in whichever capacity that was determined by the devices. Using these devices did, for a time, encourage the self-trackers to enact 'healthy' behaviours. However, this enthusiasm to track and share diminished over time. The burdens of self-tracking and the self-regulation promoted by these technologies became emotionally detrimental to their sense of wellbeing, mental and physical health. Self-trackers often perceived not maintaining 'healthy' behaviours (often due to circumstances outside of their control) as a lack of personal self-discipline. In turn, they struggled with internal contentions related to how to legitimate inactivity. This evolved into a moralisation of 'health', whereby 'health' and lifestyle choices became tied to ethical parameters of 'good' and 'bad' behaviours. In turn, self-worth became pervasively tied to data.

Self-tracking and social media as extensions of self

A key finding of this book is the role and utility of the methodological approach of this research project. The reflexive and influential role of the methodologies for the participants and the researcher was not anticipated prior to the research. The triangulation of these methods (reflexive diaries, interviews and online content) facilitated an in-depth analysis of the online and offline continuum of the digitisation of health practices and behaviours. The reflexive diaries were integral to aiding the participants' personal engagement with and understanding of their 'health' decisions, lifestyle choices and social media use. Self-tracking technologies and social media, therefore, can be seen as an extension of the self, mediating our relations, communications and the 'health' self-quantification of our being. This problematic convergence of the body and technology through health, fitness and lifestyle tracking is an inherent self-governing and self-regulatory practice that deeply permeated the participants' everyday lives. These research findings extend Lorig and Holman's (2003) argument that it is not just sufferers of chronic conditions but the everyday layperson who now embodies this dominant discourse. Health self-management, when not enacted similarly, becomes tied to personal blame (and shame) over lack of personal responsibility and poor 'health' management. Therefore, policy and the market work in tandem to construct and discursively embed the ideal neoliberal subject, a normative, fit and productive bio-citizen (Rail and Jette, 2015; Moore and Robinson, 2016). The accumulation and examination of data create extreme self-regulating pressures for self-trackers, provoking stress and anxiety, which dissolve the division between the interior and exterior of the body and blur distinctions between the biological and the social (Rose, 2013), thus normalising the 'datafication of life itself' (Ajana, 2017: 14).

The participants did feel empowered in relation to self-managing health through self-tracking data acquisition. Yet over time these (physical) activities could not always be 'lived' up to. Furthermore, the tangibility of what empowerment achieves is problematic (almost to the same extent as the term 'wellness'), as much as the abundance of data does not mean something productive is done with it or that health or fitness and overall wellness improves. For example, feeling empowered may soon turn to disempowerment if nothing can be achieved and the hoped-for 'health revolution' does not materialise. Information and ideas from social structures do not merely reflect the social world but contribute to its shape and are central to modern reflexivity. Therefore, interestingly, interpretations and rationalisations for these 'journeys' and 'health transformations' were incredibly subjective and often intangible. Much like the desire for 'wellness' or 'increasing wellbeing', this goal-driven attainment turns into a continuous and never-ending neoliberal cycle of intention, empowerment, data acquisition, goals achieved (or not) and repeat!

Interestingly, the methodological approach of this book also became an integral tool for the participants to understand 'health' decisions and practices, expanding their conceptualisations and influencing future posts, diary entries and subsequent 'health' behaviours. At times this self-analytical reflexivity was uncomfortable reading, for it highlighted their troublesome and problematic relationships with their 'health', bodies and lifestyles, particularly around obsessive and compulsive behaviours of 'over-exercising' and disordered eating practices. Many participants recognised they had 'unhealthy' relationships with how they perceived their bodies and low self-esteem and embodied self-policing regulation over their lifestyles and 'health'-related behaviours, which frequently dictated what they were and were not allowed to do. This regulation discourse was deeply embedded in their sense of moral self. To enact certain 'healthy' behaviours was to be a 'good' person. When they 'slip out' of regulatory regimes, even due to external or uncontrollable factors in their lives (stress, ill health, injury, time constraints and so on), participants felt deeply ashamed and their perception of self was of a 'bad', undisciplined individual. As Cederstrom and Spicer (2015: 5) argue, wellness is not a choice but a 'moral obligation', and the same can be said of how individuals perceive and manage their health in data-sharing spheres. Lifestyle, diet and the body became frequently tailored around the desired aesthetics and specific etiquettes of certain platforms and, most importantly, what was determined as visually pleasing on social media.

Whilst the data supported existing literature on the potential for a self-tracking utopia in relation to data acquisition and 'health' improvement, this research extends and critiques some of these arguments. The participants did often subscribe to discourses of 'self-betterment' through self-tracking, in whatever capacity that could be achieved. However, 'good health' was embodied through simple acquisition and representation of data, often over their sense of personal gratification or achievement, regardless of any improvements or achievements made. The self-trackers exhibited sceptical stances towards the efficacy and accuracy of the technologies. Yet, interestingly, this did not deter their engagement, ongoing use and self-surveillance. Self-surveying through self-tracking does not equate to 'optimal' or better 'health', for the mechanical measuring of input and output parameters promoted within self-tracking practices and categorisation became de-humanising and created reductive notions of 'health'. Users conform to a model of 'health' that advocates that, with or without technology, better 'health' is achievable only through individual bio-political governance via self-surveillance and self-regulation via data acquisition. This can be best exemplified through the input versus output discourse of health, whereby participants gamify what they consume versus their physical expenditure or exercise to effectively self-govern and regulate their health and self-improvement. These individual, technological and state level bio-political rationalities become prevalent considerations and motivations for participants to 'gamify' their health as a tool for managing individual health.

The behavioural economics of technology 'addiction'

Social media and self-tracking are platforms designed to notify and 'nudge' users to share content, like, comment and scroll. Therefore, as I conclude my findings from the research analysed in this book, it is worth coming back to the role of behavioural economics in how we engage with these platforms to consider how we might assert more agency and control with these persuasive tools of health management in our everyday life. As I have discussed in earlier chapters, 'Behavioural economics offers a means to encourage more optimal behaviour without inducing the resistance and reluctance often associated with restrictive policies' (Johnson et al, 2012: 500). And yet on social media we often find ourselves in compulsive scrolling cycles, as is identified now by a wealth of literature, including this book. Choice architecture enables a discourse and practical analysis to understand how behavioural economics is designed to keep our engagement and attention online. Thaler and Sunstein (2009: 6–8) highlight that 'setting default options (...) can have huge effects on outcomes (...) attempting to move people in directions that will make their lives better'. For example, health apps and digital devices encourage users to set and meet health goals, for example the Apple alarm + sleep cycle tracker and the Nike running app prompting users to share their jogging routes. Aside from the 'community surveillance' effect, there are many design techniques and mechanics found in healthcare apps that incorporate gamification elements to create persuasion and more instant gratification. However, as argued throughout the book, this research illustrates how these nudges and choice architecture to prompt certain health-related behaviours do not always mean 'healthier' outcomes, nor are these nudges or directions neutral.

> It is legitimate for choice architects to try to influence people's behavior in order to make their lives longer, healthier, and better. In other words, we argue for self-conscious efforts, by institutions in the private sector and also by government, to steer people's choices in directions that will improve their lives. (Thaler and Sunstein, 2009: 5)

Are these nudging interventions actually beneficial for individual health? For healthcare companies the benefits might be personalised health experiences, targeted insurance pricing and gamification opportunities. However, for the self-tracker or user the benefits are far more complex, with many unanticipated consequences, for example, a stark rise in the 'worried well' and those seeking prevention with increasing levels of anxiety related to the maintenance of their health rather than problem-solving health issues. With choice architecture on digital platforms, we will always be mediating between encouragement and coercion, never forgetting the attention economy that underpins these business models and metrics of engagement. The app may be helping the user achieve their individual goals, but the shame inflicted upon the user when they couldn't achieve a goal could be considered coercive. My research identified that persuasive computing leads to controlling human behaviour where users rely more on quantitative measures over qualitative ones – personal experiences – and emotions are discarded with an overfocus on data acquisition. As my research has shown, this does not always help to achieve health goals because it burdens individuals with a relentless push towards self-tracking. Other key findings that illustrate that relationships with self-tracking tools have become unhealthy are pushing your body according to the device rather than running a certain distance because you want to, potentially running further so you can capture the ideal image to represent your run for social media sharing. Then it is more about the performative element than the run itself, which is no bad thing unless the social media sharing becomes tied towards personal gratification through the acquisition of likes and comments, you feel guilty when you don't track or don't exercise even if mentally or physically you don't feel up to it or you start to focus more on the acquisition of data over how a run made you feel. These are some key signs the relationship with your self-tracker is becoming unhealthy.

Social media feeds us content based upon our previous likes, follows and engagement; this personalises what we see and what we don't see. Personalisation on social media is designed to become an echo-chamber of affirmation, reinforcing our views, to keep us scrolling. The obsessive yet mesmerising practice of surveillance of others can also lead to the same compulsive traits of documenting and sharing the participants' own lives. This 'gamification of health' can thus be understood as both a tool for play and health management through technology, which also generates ideological considerations related to extending mortality and preventing death. Social media is a surveillance tool – a visual archive for our personal and professional lives and a tool of visibility to watch others as well as for surveillance by tech companies, third parties and the state analysing our data. Surveillance via data is highly valuable, and it is important to remember our attention and digital traces are a big economy.

The participants in this study found that the only way they felt they could reject the 'addictive hold' these social media and self-tracking practices had over their lives was to detox, which referred to deleting the application for a period of time or quitting altogether. This research also highlights the challenges with the boundaries that constitute such 'addictions' (Turel et al, 2011), as well as the appropriate language and clinical terminology used to describe these behaviours and neuro-physiological states, as these are not yet agreed upon (Lortie and Guitton, 2013). The distinction between an addiction (the indulgence of which brings pleasure) and a compulsion (the indulgence of which merely brings relief from restless anxiety) (Alter, 2017), for example, blurs linguistic and psychiatric boundaries with these technologies. In these research findings, digital detox referred to behaviour modification, offline periods and regulatory and disciplinary time management with screen-free times. It also referred to device or technology management via deleting apps and platforms, muting notifications and reverting to analogue methods of entertainment (reading books, for example).

Digital detox, as a concept and a practice, however, relies upon the oft-discussed discourse of responsibilisation, which keeps rearing its head as a framework within the research findings in this book. This responsibalisation becomes associated with neoliberal practices encouraging individuals to manage health risks (Johnson et al, 2012: 500); if they don't take precautions, they become in some sense irresponsible. The problem with conversations around responsibilisation and digital detox is that they do not always highlight the role of platform capitalism and technology as agents of control. Are we addicted to the technology or platform itself or are we drawn into the endless information flow enabled by the digital society? Yes, digital detox can also be considered as a self-optimising method used to create a healthier lifestyle but what we must do with digital detox is to focus not on the technology itself, nor on which media technologies are being abstained from, but rather on what we realise we have lost in the process of being saturated by the technology. Digital detox will not necessarily make you happier or increase your productivity; individuals should identify their own problems, or personal and emotional voids, through the process of digital detox. So, what can we do to wade through the persuasive and coercive choice architecture of self-tracking and social media platforms? Is there a solution? Listen to your body – trust how you feel and your human instinct over a device's nudges, or your desire for personal data capture. Think about why you are tracking and whether it is necessary for your fitness and running goals. If so, ensure that you are physically and mentally listening to your body instead of the guidance, nudges or notifications of an application/tracker. Finally, remember these platforms want your attention as much as and for as long as possible.

Future research

The digital economy largely relies upon information technology, data and the internet for their business models. Throughout the analyses in this book, I have demonstrated how data has become a currency for citizens and consumers to pay for free communication and services via digital platforms – a now-accepted trade-off as members of a digital society: 'As consumers, we are presented with a cornucopia of on-demand services and with the promise of a network of connected devices that cater to our every whim' (Srnicek, 2017: 1). Capitalism has turned to data as one way to maintain economic growth, which is dependent on platforms to generate it. van Dijck argues (2014: 1) that this is illustrative of the widespread secular belief in dataism, which is 'so successful, because masses of people – naively or unwittingly – trust their personal information to corporate platforms'. As I discussed in Chapter 2, 'Understanding Our Bodies through Datafication', the amount of data about health that can be collected from everyday activity has grown rapidly in recent years; advertisers are predicting and marketing health, wellbeing and fitness products to us recommended by algorithms predicting our next health-related purchase interest. Digital phenotyping refers to the analysis of our personal data to infer our personal health status, for example, by social media analytics companies rather than traditional healthcare settings such as a GP surgery or hospital (Ada Lovelace Institute, 2020). Similarly, this data can be repurposed and used for purposes unrelated or not directly related to healthcare, such as risk assessments for insurance premiums (Ada Lovelace Institute, 2020).

Ideals of 'data philanthropy', sharing data for the public good and public health, have been accelerated by economic structures of data capitalism whereby personal health data is now a capitalist commodity. With COVID-19 as the first pandemic of the algorithmic age (Ada Lovelace Institute, 2020), this is becoming increasingly normalised, with widespread surveillance of population health through international implementation of contact tracing applications. Digital contact tracing and immunity certification have dominated public discourse, and data-driven technologies, such as AI-assisted chest scans and centralised public health datastores, have been central to many nations' responses to the virus. The data these innovations draw on is largely collected from medical settings, but many types of data that aren't commonly associated with health have been crucial to understanding the impact of COVID-19. Importantly, within these practices of state and public health surveillance, as well as personalisation as a mode of surveillance, we are being risk profiled. Rather than illegal or criminal behaviour, surveillance for health risk management has now become a part of daily law-enforced citizen responsibilisation practice for individuals and public health – a true embodiment of the digital health self.

Now, I imagine there are very few people who do not care about personal and public health, particularly in response to managing COVID-19 and beyond. However, these ideals of data philanthropy to safeguard public health are not the key issue here. The notion of trust, from citizens, becomes a contentious deliberation as individuals' faith is extended to be managed by the state and public institutions such as law enforcement and healthcare, who have access to our (meta)data. This comes from a place of reliance on, and automation of, control and monitoring via digital technologies and normalising large-scale surveillance systems. Several researchers argue that the adoption of digital contact tracing applications could lead to the economic exploitation of private data and may also create a mass electronic surveillance system (Martinez-Martin et al, 2020; Vaithianathan et al, 2020), despite high acceptability rates among the UK population (74.8 per cent of the participants within the sample are in favour of voluntary digital tracing and 68.8 per cent are in favour of automatic applications) (Altmann et al, 2020). Datafication also creates increasingly comprehensive and quantified renderings of health, creating the conditions for disempowerment and providing unprecedented opportunities to monitor and influence people. What this means is that a wealth and variety of public and private actors, such as governments, healthcare systems, the tech industry, employers and insurers, can now have access to, make inferences from and repurpose our health and personal data for a multitude of different incentives. Security and privacy issues often pose contradictory demands, leading to ambivalent legal definitions, as legitimate means for dataveillance. Citizens' groups rightly call for clear-cut policies that guard privacy and balance it off with security. Bringing legal definitions in tune with advanced technological apparatuses is just one pivotal step in the effort to rebuild trust and, perhaps most importantly, transparency, for users and for citizens.

Health is no longer situated at the responsibility, or inhabitation of the individual, or between the individual or the healthcare provider as two-way transactional relationship. Health is now repurposed and inferenced using so many different life domains through different digital trails, meaning boundaries of what is or is not data about health are no longer clear (Ada Lovelace Institute, 2020). Data is the glue that takes separate parts of personal healthcare and makes them into a whole, ensuring current legal definitions and practical frameworks for governing health data need to move in line with these digital evolutions (Ada Lovelace Institute, 2020). For these practices, mining and monetization of health and wellness in the digital economy change our experience of what 'healthiness is in everyday life. Furthermore, the digital economy shapes understandings and practices of health and wellness now and in the future both for individuals and for the digital society as a whole. In other words, we must as users, individuals, patients and citizens be acutely aware now that our everyday digital traces are mined and profiled to the extent that it is conceivable that 'all data is health data' (Warzel, 2019). Therefore, it is always worth recognising that our digital (health) behaviour is now monetised, and recommendation algorithms and targeted advertising are often one step ahead of our choices. The avocation of digital health tools from tech giants, and within public health promotional policy, particularly during COVID-19 and beyond, is deserving of urgent analysis.

The digital health self

Monitoring and managing our health via self-tracking tools and social media are not just about the technology but rather about what it means when we use these technologies and the physical, mental or emotional changes that occur as a response to political, economic and socio-economic underpinnings; I conceptualise this as the embodiment of the digital health self. For even when technology is removed or resisted in these surveillant and self-tracking cultures, regulation of the body with or without the tools and technologies of the self is still prevalent, preventative and self-policing in the mind of the users. This dualism then, where the mind is conceived as holding a powerful condition over bodily matter (Moore and Robinson, 2016), situated the participants as actors who must 'control' and take responsibility for their biology. Problematically, this removed their recognition of physical impossibilities, as the discourses that surround these technologies remove subjectivity and the important medical and biological recognition that all bodies do not behave or perform in the same way. Nor do all bodies have the same capacities and will 'transform' through calculated or measured intervention, no matter how much one person may want to 'better' or 'optimise' themselves. This perspective is forming a new social shaping and understanding of bodily capacities. The reduction of the body to data or technological interpretation is shaped and formed by the meanings in which they are enmeshed. Yet these embodiments engage with shaping processes and realities provided only by using these technologies alone.

The engagement with self-tracking practices leads users to overvalue the data representations of their 'health' and their bodies. Problematically, representations of 'good health' on social media were the focus for many users, often over undertaking 'healthier' activities. These representations of 'health' frequently stand in for users' actual physical 'health' (improvements), without motivating them to 'get healthier'. This is hugely problematic, if over time representations of 'health' rather than actual health outcomes become the main priority for self-trackers who share. In turn, we may 'trust the machine's representation more than our own memories' (Rettberg, 2018: 29). Habits related to posting and self-tracking can be conceived as governable in these data-sharing cultures. Self-tracking makes 'past and current events equally knowable. The very ideas of "past" and "present" in relation to personal information are in danger of evaporating. The past is on the surface' (Allen, 2008: 62). The role and nature of human memory to be forgetful or to omit certain things may protect us from traumatic past events. This draws attention to the complexities of human senses and capabilities, one that a computer or self-tracking technology could never imitate. Biological memory serves us well, but it is highly selective and fallible (Allen, 2008). With social media and self-tracking technologies, what happened in the past and what happened today are now equally 'knowable'. Yet memory and data are two very different things. Data is limited, while memory is complex, supportive and adapts to suit the needs of every individual. Data is only individual in so much as it is specific to you. The human mind, memory, senses, instinct and intuition can and do tell us more than data. The participants in this research celebrated the capacities for the human mind to provide voluntary amnesia from traumatic events, while data representations drew painful attention to them. As Allen (2008: 55–56) astutely observes:

> Memory can be a very good thing, but it can also encourage harmfully dredging up or revisiting past conduct. Surveillance can also be a very good thing, but it turns into a social evil when it trains watchful, spying eyes needlessly and hurtfully.

Nostalgia is our own invention (Foucault, 1988) and yet holds powerful parameters for the 'optimal' body, providing idealised notions of 'health' and our relationship to past healthy selves and disciplinary acts. This is especially prevalent when being identified as not a reality in the present time or in the present body. Self-tracking proposes mutations in our very idea of a 'healthy life'. The pure mechanisms of our bodies and our brains have become engineer-able apparatuses. This takes us beyond the binary of the normal and the pathological. With these technologies, we routinely attempt to take our pathology into our own hands. These technologies cannot consider the non-sequential nature of ill health and disease. How then can we disregard elements that we cannot quantify or neatly capture, especially if, in turn, we increasingly limit our understanding of life itself and, within it, pathologies and 'health'?

These research findings have identified a discourse that encourages individuals to prioritise the 'maximisation' and 'optimisation' of what we have come to believe is our quality of life. Problematically, this continual management should, as it has been demonstrated, not be reduced to 'good' or 'bad' representations of 'health', nor should specific qualities and determinants of certain 'lifestyle realities' be privileged over others. These surveillant, monitoring, competitive and comparative technologies propose such binaries by nudging users through forms and tools of engagement. Even when these regulatory frames are finally resisted, and digital detoxing liberates, the technologies' presence and role are still committed in the minds of their users. These are technologies of control, over the body and mind, for when they are finally removed, they still situate their (prior) dominance and pervasive self-regulation in the present time and in the present minds of their users. These complex ensembles of knowledge, technologies, subjectivities and ethics suggest the perception, expectation and hope of a healthier, fitter, 'better' and 'optimised' future. Individual quality of life, therefore, becomes about perception and expectation as advocated by the technology. These technologies imagine the future; they force us to bring the future into the present by controlling our bodies. The digital health self manages the present body in order to produce a better 'healthier' future and demands the future body as a right and a reward for past 'health' management.

References

Aakhus, M. (2002) *Perpetual Contact: Mobile Communication, Private Talk, Public Performance*, New York: Cambridge University Press.

Abrahamse, W., Steg, L., Vlek, C. and Rothengatter, T. (2005) 'A review of intervention studies aimed at household energy conservation', *Journal of Environmental Psychology*, 25(3): 273–291, doi: 10.1016/j.jenvp.2005.08.002.

Abroms, L., Padmanabhan, N., Thaweethai, L. and Phillips, T. (2011) 'iPhone apps for smoking cessation', *American Journal of Preventive Medicine*, 40(3): 279–285.

Ada Lovelace Institute (2020) 'The Data Will See You Now' Available from: https://www.adalovelaceinstitute.org/wp-content/uploads/2020/11/The-data-will-see-you-now-Ada-Lovelace-Institute-Oct-2020.pdf [Accessed 22 February 2023].

Adam, B. (1998) *Timescapes of Modernity: The Environment and Invisible Hazards*, London: Routledge.

Adams, M. and Raisborough, J. (2008) 'Mockery and morality in popular cultural representations of the white working class', *Sociological Research Online*, 13(6): 2, doi: 10.5153/sro.1814.

Adams, S. (2012) 'Post-panoptic surveillance through healthcare rating sites', *Information, Communication & Society*, 16(2): 215–235.

Aguirre, Jr., A., Eick, V. and Reese, R. (2006) 'Introduction: neoliberal globalization, urban privatization, and resistance', *Social Justice*, 33(3): 1–5.

Ahuja, N.K. (2013) '"It feels good to be measured": clinical role-play, Walker Percy, and the tingles', *Perspectives in Biology and Medicine*, 56(3): 442–445.

Ajana, B. (2005) 'Surveillance and biopolitics', *Electronic Journal of Sociology*, 7, available from: https://www.researchgate.net/publication/236672756_Ajana_B_2005_'Surveillance_and_Biopolitics'_Electronic_Journal_of_Sociology_vol7 [Accessed 16 March 2023].

Ajana, B. (2010) 'Recombinant identities: biometrics and narrative bioethics', *Journal of Bioethical Inquiry*, 7(2): 237–258.

Ajana, B. (2012) 'Biometric citizenship', *Citizen Studies*, 16(7): 851–870.

Ajana, B. (2013) *Governing through Biometrics: The Biopolitics of Identity*, Basingstoke: Palgrave Macmillan.

Ajana, B. (2014) 'Augmented boarders: big data and the ethics of immigration control', *Journal of Information, Communication & Ethics in Society*, Special Issue: Immigration, ICT and Ethics, 13(1): 58–78.

Ajana, B. (2017) 'Digital health and the biopolitics of the quantified self', *Digital Health*, 3(1): 1–18, doi: 10.1177/2055207616689509.

Ajana, B. (2018a) 'Communal self-tracking: data philanthropy, solidarity and privacy', in B. Ajana (ed) *Self-Tracking: Empirical and Philosophical Investigations*, Cham: Palgrave Macmillan, 125–142.

Ajana, B. (ed) (2018b) *Metric Culture: Ontologies of Self-Tracking Practices*, London: Emerald Publishing.

Albrechtslund, A. (2008) 'Online social networking as participatory surveillance', *First Monday*, 13(3), Available from: http://firstmonday.org/article/view/2142/1949 [Accessed 1 June 2018].

Allan, S. (2000) *Media, Risk and Science*, Buckingham: Open University Press.

Allen, A.L. (2008) 'Dredging-up the past: lifelogging, memory and surveillance', *The University of Chicago Law Review*, 75(1): 47–74.

Alter, A. (2017) *Irresistible: Why We Can't Stop Checking, Scrolling, Clicking and Watching*, London: Random House.

Altmann, S., Milsom, L., Zillessen, H., Blasone, R., Gerdon, F., Bach, R., Kreuter, F., Nosenzo, D., Toussaert, S. and Abeler, J. (2020) 'Acceptability of app-based contact tracing for COVID-19: Cross-country survey study', *JMIR mHealth and uHealth*, 8(8): e19857.

American Psychiatric Association (2013) 'Internet gaming disorder', in American Psychiatric Association (ed) *Diagnostic and Statistical Manual of Mental Disorders*, Arlington: American Psychiatric Publishing, 795–798.

American Psychological Association (2020) *Publication Manual of the American Psychological Association*, Washington, DC: American Psychological Association.

Amir, O. and Lobel, O. (2008) 'Stumble, predict, nudge: how behavioural economics informs law and policy', *Columbia Law Review*, 108(8): 2098–2137.

Anderson, B. (1983) *Imagined Communities: Reflections on the Origin and Spread of Nationalism*, London: Verso.

Anderson, C.L., Monroy, M. and Keltner, D. (2018) 'Awe in nature heals: evidence from military veterans, at-risk youth, and college students', *Emotion (Washington, D.C.)*, 18(8): 1195–1202, doi: 10.1037/emo0000442.

Anderson, W. and Gillam, S. (2001) 'The elusive NHS consumer: 1948 to the NHS Plan', *Economic Affairs*, 12(4): 14–18.

Andersson, E. and Olson, M. (2014) 'Political participation as public pedagogy – the educational situation in young people's political conversations in social media', *Journal of Social Science Education*, 13(4): 115–126.

Andreassen, C.S., Torsheim, T., Brunborg, G.S. and Pallesen, S. (2012) 'Development of a Facebook addiction scale', *Psychological Reports*, 110(2): 501–517.

Andrejevic, M. (2015) 'Foreword', in R.E. Dubrofsky and A.M. Shoshana (eds) *Feminist Surveillance Studies*, Durham and London: Duke University Press, 1–12.

Androutsopoulos, J. (2008) 'Potentials and limitations of discourse-centred online ethnography', *Language@Internet*, 5, 9–18.

Ariely, D. (2011) 'Predictably irrational: the hidden forces that shape our decisions', Department of Health, Healthy Lives, Healthy People: Call to Action on Obesity, 10, Available from: https://www.gov.uk/government/uploads/system/uploads/attachment_data/file/134840/dh_130487.pdf [Accessed 25 May 2018].

Armour, K.M. and Chambers, F.C. (2014) ' "Sport and exercise pedagogy": the case for a new integrative sub-discipline in the field of sport and exercise sciences/kinesiology/human movement sciences', *Sport, Education and Society*, 19(7): 855–868.

Armstrong, D. (1995) 'The rise of surveillance medicine', *Sociology of Health & Illness*, 17(3): 393–404.

Arnaut, K. (2012) 'Super-diversity: elements of an emerging perspective', *Diversities*, 14(2): 1–16.

Ayo, N. (2011) 'Understanding health promotion in a neoliberal climate and the making of health conscious citizens', *Critical Public Health*, 22(1): 1–7.

Banner, O. (2012) 'Patient 2.0: bio-mediated illness and digital intimacies', in J. Rak and M. Poletti (eds) *Identity Technologies*, Madison: University of Wisconsin Press, 196–216.

Barad, K. (2003) 'Posthumanist performativity: toward an understanding of how matter comes to matter', *Signs*, 28(3): 801–831, https://doi.org/10.1086/345321.

Barad, K. (2007) *Meeting the Universe Halfway: Quantum Physics and the Entanglement of Matter and Meaning*, Durham, NC, and London: Duke University Press.

Barad, K. (2018) Kleinman, A. Interview with Karen Barad 'Intra-Actions'. Available at: https://www.academia.edu/1857617/_Intra_actions_Interview_of_Karen_Barad_by_Adam_Kleinmann_ [Accessed 23 February 2023].

Barthes, R. (1957) *Mythologies*, Paris: Editions du Seuil.

Bartky, S.L. (1990) *Femininity and Domination: Studies in the Phenomenology of Oppression*, New York: Routledge.

Bassett, C. (2012) 'The real estate of the trained-up self: (or is this England?)', in R. Wilken and G. Goggin (eds) *Mobile Technology and Place*, New York: Routledge, 104–122.

Baum, F. (2008) 'The Commission on the Social Determinants of Health: reinventing health promotion for the twenty-first century?', *Critical Public Health*, 18(4): 457–466.

Bauman, Z. (2000) *Liquid Modernity*, Cambridge: Polity Press.

Baumeister, R.F. and Leary, M.R. (1995) 'The need to belong: desire for interpersonal attachments as a fundamental human motivation', *Psychological Bulletin*, 117(3): 497–529, doi: 10.1037/0033-2909.117.3.497.

Baym, N.K. (2010) *Personal Connections in the Digital Age*, Cambridge: Polity Press.
BBC News (2020) 'Love Island stars and influencers paid to promote Test and Trace', 31 August. Available at: https://www.bbc.co.uk/news/business-53968222 [Accessed 22 February 2023].
BCC Research (Analyst Andrew McWilliams) (2017) 'Health self-monitoring: technologies and global markets', Available from: https://www.bccresearch.com/market-research/healthcare/health-self-monitoring-technologies-markets-report-hlc185b.html [Accessed 25 May 2020].
Beard, A. (ed) (2000) *The Language of Politics*, London: Routledge.
Beato, G. (2012) 'The quantified self', *Reason*, 43(8): 18–20.
Beaulieu, A. (2007) 'Mediating ethnography: objectivity and the making of ethnographies of the internet', *Social Epistemology*, 18(2–3): 139–163.
Beck, U. (1992) *Risk Society: Towards a New Modernity*, London: SAGE.
Beck, U. and Beck-Gersheim, E. (2001) *Individualization: Institutionalized Individualism and Its Social and Political Consequences*, London: SAGE.
Beck, U., Giddens, A. and Lash, S. (1994) *Reflexive Modernisation: Politics, Tradition and Aesthetics in the Modern Social Order*, Cambridge: Polity Press.
Beer, D. (2008) 'Researching a confessional society', *International Journal of Market Research*, 50(5): 619.
Beer, D. (2009) 'Power through the algorithm? Participatory web cultures and the technological unconscious', *New Media & Society*, 11(6): 985–1002.
Beer, D. (2016) *Metric Power*, London: Palgrave Macmillan.
Beer, D. and Burrows, R. (2007) 'Sociology and, of and in web 2.0: some initial considerations', *Sociological Research Online*, 12(5): np.
Beer, D. and Burrows, R. (2010) 'Consumption, prosumption and participatory web cultures: an introduction', *Journal of Consumer Culture*, 10(1): 3–12.
Benjamin, W. (1973) 'The work of art in the age of mechanical reproduction', in W. Benjamin (ed) *Illuminations*, London: Fontana, 211–244.
Bentham, J. (2011). The Panopticon Writings [edition unavailable], London: Verso . Available from https://www.perlego.com/book/3785689/the-panopticon-writings-pdf (Original work published 1791).
Bernstein, B. (2001) 'From pedagogies to knowledges', in A. Morais, I. Neves, B. Davies and H. Daniels (eds) *Towards a Sociology of Pedagogy. The Contribution of Basil Bernstein to Research*, New York: Peter Lang, 363–368.
Berry, C., Harbord, J. and Moore, R.O. (2013) *Public Space, Media Space*, Basingstoke: Palgrave Macmillan.
Berry, D. (2012) *Life in Code and Software: Mediated Life in a Complex Computational Ecology*, London: Open Humanities Press.
Berry, D.M. and Michael, D. (eds) (2015) *Postdigital Aesthetics: Art, Computation and Design*, Basingstoke: Palgrave Macmillan.
Berson, J. (2015) *Computable Bodies: Instrumented Life and the Human Somatic Niche*, London: Bloomsbury.

Beskorovajnov, W., F. Dorre, G. Hartung, A. Koch, J. Muller-Quade, and T. Strufe. (2020) 'ConTra Corona: contact tracing against the coronavirus by bridging the centralized-decentralized divide for stronger privacy', IACR Cryptology ePrint Archive 2020: 505, Available from: https://eprint.iacr.org/2020/505.pdf [Accessed 16 March 2023].

Besley, T. and Peters, M.A. (2007) *Subjectivity & Truth: Foucault, Education, and the Culture of Self* (Vol. 303), New York: Peter Lang.

Best, K. (2010) 'Living in the control society: surveillance, users and digital screen technologies', *International Journal of Cultural Studies*, 13(1): 5–24.

Bijker, W. and Law, J. (eds) (1992) *Shaping Technology/Building Society: Studies in Sociotechnical Change*, Cambridge, MA: MIT Press.

Billig, M. (1999) 'The language of critical discourse analysis: the case of normalisation', in R. Wodak and M. Meyer (eds) *Methods of Critical Discourse Analysis: History, Theory and Methodology*, London: SAGE, 23–41.

Blair, A. (2003) 'Reading strategies for coping with information overload ca 1550-1700', *Journal of the History of Ideas*, 64: 11–28.

Blommaert, J. (2007) 'On scope and depth in linguistic ethnography', *Journal of Sociolinguistics*, 11(5): 682–688.

Blommaert, J. (2013) *Ethnography, Superdiversity and Linguistic Landscapes. Chronicles of Complexity*, Bristol: Multilingual Matters.

Blower, L. (2016) 'It's "because I am a woman": realizing identity to reconstruct identity for the female autobiographical inquiry', *Convergence: The Journal of Research into New Media Technologies*, 22: 88–101.

Bode, M. and Kristensen, D.B. (2016) 'The digital doppelgänger within. A study on self-tracking and the quantified self movement', in D. Bajde and R. Canniford (eds) *Assembling Consumption*, New York: Routledge, 119–134.

Boellstorff, T., Nardi, B., Taylor, T.L. and Pearce, C. (2012) *Ethnography and Virtual Worlds: A Handbook of Method*, Princeton: Princeton University Press.

Bogard, W. (1996) *The Simulation of Surveillance: Hyper Control in Telematic Societies*, Cambridge: Cambridge University Press.

Bossewitch, J. and Sinnreich, A. (2013) 'The end of forgetting: strategic agency beyond the panopticon', *New Media & Society*, 15(2): 224–242.

Bottles, K. (2012) 'Will the quantified self movement take off in health care?', *Physician Executive*, 38(5): 74–75.

Bourdieu, P. (1984) *Distinction: A Social Critique of the Judgement of Taste*, London: Routledge.

Bowden, M. (2012) 'The measured man', *The Atlantic Magazine*, Available from: http://www.theatlantic.com/magazine/archive/2012/07/the-measured-man/309018/ [Accessed 25 May 2018].

boyd, d. (2008a) 'How can qualitative internet researchers define the boundaries of their projects: a response to Christine Hine', in A.N. Markham and K.N. Baum (eds) *Internet Inquiry: Conversations about Method*, Los Angeles: SAGE, 26–32.

boyd, d. (2008b) 'Why youth ♥ social network sites', in D. Buckingham (ed) *Youth, Identity, and Digital Media*, Cambridge, MA: MIT Press, 119–142.

boyd, d. (2010a) 'Privacy and publicity in the context of big data', WWW 2010, Raleigh, North Carolina, 29 April, Available from: http://www.danah.org/papers/talks/2010/WWW2010.html [Accessed 12 July 2014].

boyd, d. (2010b) 'Social network sites as networked publics: affordances, dynamics, and implications', in Z. Papacharissi (ed) *A Networked Self: Identity, Community, and Culture on Social Network* Sites, London: Routledge, 39–58.

boyd, d. (2014) *It's Complicated: The Social Lives of Networked Teens*, New Haven: Yale University Press.

boyd, d. and Ellison, N.B. (2007) 'Social network sites: definition, history, and scholarship', *Journal of Computer-Mediated Communication*, 13(1): 210–230.

boyd, d. and Hargittai, E. (2010) 'Facebook privacy settings: who cares?', *First Monday*, 15(8), Available from: http://firstmonday.org/article/view/3086/2589 [Accessed 1 June 2018].

boyd, d. and Crawford, K. (2012) 'Critical questions for big data: provocations for a cultural, technological, and scholarly phenomenon', *Information, Communication & Society*, 15(5): 662–679.

Boyne, R. (2000) 'Post-panopticon', *Economy and Society*, 29(2): 285–307.

Brabazon, T. (2015) 'Facing off: theorizing over-sharing and under-reading', *Online Journal of Communication and Media Technologies*, 5(1): 57–73.

Braidotti, R. (2005) 'Affirming the affirmative: on nomadic affectivity', *Rhizomes*, 11–12.

Braidotti, R. (2006) *Transpositions*, Cambridge and Malden: Polity Press.

Braidotti, R. (2019) 'A Theoretical Framework for the Critical Posthumanities', *Theory, Culture & Society*, 36(6): 31–61. https://doi.org/10.1177/0263276418771486.

Brandt, A. and Rozin, P. (eds) (1997) *Morality and Health*, London: Routledge.

Braudel, F. (1980) 'History and the social sciences: the longue duree', in E. Braudel (ed) and S. Matthews trans) *Braudel on History*, London: Wiedenfeld and Nicolson, np.

Brenner, N. and Theodore, N. (2002) 'Cities and geographies of "actually existing neoliberalism"', *Antipode*, 34: 349–379.

Brenner, N., Peck, J. and Theodore, N. (2006) 'Introduction: neoliberal globalization, urban privatization, and resistance', *Social Justice*, 33(3): 1–5.

Brewer, J.D. (2000) *Ethnography*, Buckingham: Open University Press.

Briggs, C.L. (1986) *Learning How to Ask. A Sociolinguistic Appraisal of the Role of the Interview in Social Science Research*, Cambridge: Cambridge University Press.

Brighenti, A.M. (2010) 'On territorology: towards a general science of territory', *Theory, Culture & Society*, 27(1): 52–72.

Brin, D. (1998) *The Transparent Society: Will Technology Force Us to Choose between Privacy and Freedom?*, Cambridge, MA: Perseus Book Group.

Brown, W. (2003) 'American nightmare: neoliberalism, neoconservatism and de-democratisation', *Political Theory*, 34(6): 690–714.

Brown, W. (2005) 'Neoliberalism and the end of liberal democracy', in W. Brown (ed) *Edgework: Critical Essays on Knowledge and Politics*, Woodstock: Princeton University Press, 37–59.

Browne, S. (2015) *Dark Matters: On the Surveillance of Blackness*, Los Angeles: Duke University Press.

Brownsword, R. (2002) *Rights, Regulation, and the Technological Revolution*, Oxford: Oxford University Press.

Brownsword, R. (2004) 'What the world needs now: techno-regulation, human rights and human dignity', in R. Brownsword (ed) *Human Rights*, Oxford: Hart Publishing, 3–9.

Bruns, A. and Schmidt, J. (2011) 'Produsage: a closer look at continuing developments', *New Review of Hypermedia and Multimedia*, 17(1): 3–7.

Bryman, A. (2001) *Social Research Methods*, Oxford: Oxford University Press.

Burchell, G. (1993) 'Liberal government and techniques of the self', *Economy and Society*, 22(3): 267–282.

Butler, J. (1997) *Excitable Speech: On the Politics of the Performative*, London: Routledge.

Butler, J. (2005) *Giving an Account of Oneself*, New York: Fordham University Press.

Butt, C. (2012) 'For some, appiness is self-quantified', *Technology – The Sydney Morning Herald*, 30 December, Available from: http://www.smh.com.au/technology/technology-news/for-some-appiness-is-selfquantified-20121229–2c0b3.html [Accessed 16 October 2015].

Butterfield, A.D. (2012) 'Ethnographic assessment of quantified self meetup groups', QuantifiedSelf.com, Available from: http://quantifiedself.com/wp-content/uploads/2012/05/Adam-Project-Report-5-17.pdf [Accessed 13 June 2015].

Buyx, A. and Prainsack, B. (2012) 'Lifestyle related diseases and individual responsibility through the prism of solidarity', *Clinical Ethics*, 7(2): 79–85.

Cacioppo, J.T. et al (2002) 'Loneliness and health: potential mechanisms', *Psychosomatic Medicine*, 64(3): 407–417, doi: 10.1097/00006842-200205000-00005.

Calhoun, J.B. (1962) 'Population density and social pathology', *Scientific American*, 206(2): 139–148.

Campbell, D. (2010) 'How to get public health policy right: listen to the public', *The Guardian*, 18 August, Available from: http://www.guardian.co.uk/society/joepublic/2010/aug/18/public-should-lead-public-health-policy [Accessed 25 May 2020].

Cancer Research UK (2017) 'Cancer research highlights: a patient's pick', Available from: http://scienceblog.cancerresearchuk.org/2017/12/20/2017-cancer-research-highlights-a-patients-pick/ [Accessed 25 May 2018].

Canguilhem, G. (ed) (1978) *On the Normal and the Pathological*, Studies in the History of Modern Science, Dordrecht: Springer.

Canguilhem, G. (2012) *Forms of Living: Writings on Medicine*, New York: Fordham University Press.

Carmichael, A. (2010) 'Why I stopped tracking', QuantifiedSelf.com, Available from: http://quantifiedself.com/2010/04/why-i-stopped-tracking/11 [Accessed 25 May 2018].

Caron-Flinterman, J.F., Broerse, J.E., Bunders, J.F. (2005) 'The experiential knowledge of patients: a new resource for biomedical research?', *Social Science and Medicine*, 60(11): 2575–2584. doi: 10.1016/j.socscimed.2004.11.023.

Casey, A., Goodyear, V.A. and Armour, K.M. (2017) 'Rethinking the relationship between pedagogy, technology and learning in health and physical education', *Sport, Education and Society*, 22: 288–304.

Casper, M. and Morrison, D. (2010) 'Medical sociology and technology: critical engagements', *Journal of Health and Social Behaviour*, 51(1): S120–S132.

Cederstrom, C. and Spicer, A. (2015) *The Wellness Syndrome*, London: John Wiley & Sons.

Cheney-Lippold, J. (2011) 'A new algorithmic identity: soft bio-politics and the modulation of control', *Theory, Culture & Society*, 28(6): 164–181.

Cheng, V.J. (2004) *Inauthentic: The Anxiety over Culture and Identity*, New Jersey: Rutgers University Press.

Chou, Y.Y.S., Prestin, A., Lyons, C. and Wen, K.Y. (2013) 'Web 2.0 for health promotion: reviewing the current evidence', *American Journal of Public Health*, 103(1): e9–e18, Available from: http://ajph.aphapublications.org/doi/abs/10.2105/AJPH.2012.301071?prevSearch=we+b+2.0&searchHistoryKey=.& [Accessed 5 October 2015].

Christakis, N. and Fowler, J. (2009) *Connected: The Surprising Power of Our Social Networks*, New York: Hachette.

Christensen, L. (2013) 'Big brother health or mindful living? Quantified-self organiser Steve Dean on the difference between self-tracking and surveillance', *Vanity Fair*, 8 January, Available from: http://www.vanityfair.com/online/daily/2013/01/quantified-self-organizer-steven-dean-interview-surveillance [Accessed 5 October 2015].

Chrysanthou, M. (2002) 'Transparency and selfhood: utopia and the informed body', *Social Science & Medicine*, 54(3): 469–479.

Clarke, R. (1988) 'Information technology and dataveillance', *Communications of the ACM*, 31(5): 498–512.

Clifford, J. and Marcus, G.E. (1998) *Writing Culture: The Poetics & Politics of Ethnography*, Berkeley: University of California Press.

Clough, T.P. (2010) 'The case of sociology: governmentality and methodology', *Critical Inquiry*, 36(4): 627–641.

Cobley, P. (2006) 'A brief note on dialogue', in S. Petrilli (ed) *Victoria Welby and the Science of Signs, Significs, Semiotics, and the Philosophy of Language*, Bari: Edizioni dal Sud, 13–20.

Cockroft, R. and Cockroft, S. (1992) *Persuading People: An Introduction to Rhetoric*, London: Macmillan.

Coggon, J. (2012) *What Makes Health Public? A Critical Evaluation of Moral, Legal, & Political Claims in Public Health*, Cambridge: Cambridge University Press.

Cohen, S. (1985) *Visions of Social Control*, Cambridge: Polity Press.

Coiera, E. (2013) 'Social networks, social media, and social diseases', *British Medical Journal*, 346: f3007, doi: https://doi.org/10.1136/bmj.f3007.

Coleman, G.E. (2010) 'Ethnographic approaches to digital media', *Annual Review of Anthropology*, 39: 487–505.

Conor, L. (2004) *The Spectacular Modern Woman: Feminine Visibility in the 1920s*, Bloomington: Indiana University Press.

Conquergood, D. (1991) 'Rethinking ethnography: Towards a critical cultural politics', *Communication Monographs*, 58:2, 179–194, DOI:10.1080/03637759109376222.

Cote, M. (2011) 'Learning to immaterial labour 2.0: Facebook and social networks', in M. Peters and E. Bulut (eds) *Cognitive Capitalism, Education and Digital Labour*, New York: Peter Lang, 169–193.

Cote, M. (2014) 'The pre-historic turn? Networked new media, mobility and the body', in A. Vivildia, J. Nerone, V. Mayer, S. Mazzarella and R. Parameswaran (eds) *The International Encyclopedia of Media Studies*, Vol. 6, London: Blackwell 130–140.

Coughlan, R. (2006) 'The socio-politics of technology and innovation: problematizing the "caring" in healthcare?', *Social Theory & Health*, 4(4): 334–352.

Couldry, N. (2003) *Media Rituals: A Critical Approach*, London: Routledge.

Couldry, N. (2012) *Media, Society, World: Social Theory and Digital Media Practice*, Cambridge: Polity Press.

Couldry, N., Fotopoulou, A. and Dickens, L. (2016) 'Real social analytics: a contribution towards a phenomenology of a digital world', *The British Journal of Sociology*, 67(1): 118–137.

Coveney, J. (1998) 'The government and ethics of health promotion: the importance of Michel Foucault', *Health Education Research*, 13(3): 459–468.

Crawford, R. (1977) 'You are dangerous to your health: the ideology and politics of victim blaming', *International Journal of Health Services*, 7(4): 663–680.

Crawford, R. (1980) 'Healthism and the medicalisation of everyday life', *International Journal of Health Care Services*, 10(3): 365–388.

Crawford, R. (2006) 'Health as meaningful practice', *Health: An Interdisciplinary Journal for the Social Study of Health, Illness and Medicine*, 10(4): 401–420.

Crawshaw, P. (2012) 'Governing at a distance: social marketing and the (bio) politics of responsibility', *Social Science & Medicine*, 74(1): 200–207.

Crawshaw, P. (2013) 'Public health policy and the behavioural turn: the case of social marketing', *Critical Social Policy*, 33(4): 616–637.

Crouch, C. (2011) *The Strange Non-death of Neoliberalism*, Cambridge: Polity Press.

Dandeker, C. (1990) *Surveillance, Power, and Modernity: Bureaucracy and Discipline from 1700 to the Present Day*, Cambridge: Polity Press.

Daston, L. and Galison, P. (2010) *Objectivity*, New York: Zone Books.

Davies, P.C.W. (1982) *The Accidental Universe*, Cambridge: Cambridge University Press.

Davies, W. (2015) *The Limits of Neoliberalism: Authority, Sovereignty and the Logic of Competition*, London: SAGE.

Davies, W. (2016) *The Happiness Industry*, London: Verso.

Davin, S. (2005) 'Public medicine: the reception of a medical drama', in M. King and K. Watson (eds) *Representing Health: Discourses of Health and Illness in the Media*, Basingstoke: Palgrave Macmillan.

Davis, S.E. (2018) 'Objectification, sexualization, and misrepresentation: social media and the college experience', *Social Media + Society*, 4(3). https://doi.org/10.1177/2056305118786727.

De Certeau, M. (1984) *The Practice of Everyday Life*, Berkeley: University of California Press.

De Lange, M. (2013) 'The smart city you love to hate: exploring the role of affect in hybrid urbanism', Conference Paper, The Hybrid City II: Subtle Revolutions, 23–25 May, Athens, Greece, Available from: http://www.bijt.org/wordpress/wp-content/uploads/2006/01/Michiel_de_Lange-The-smart-city-you-love-to-hate-exploring-the-role-of-affect_Hybrid_City-Athens_styled_edit-v2.pdf [Accessed 1 June 2018].

De Lauretis, T. (1987) *Technologies of Gender: Essays on Theory, Film, and Fiction*, Bloomington: Indiana University Press.

De Maria, A.N. (2012) 'Self-quantification of health and fitness', *Journal of the American College of Cardiology*, 60(16): 1574–1575.

De Souza, E. and Silva, A. (2006) 'From cyber to hybrid: mobile technologies as interfaces of hybrid spaces', *Space and Culture*, 9(3): 261–278.

De Souza, E., Silva, A. and Sutko, D.M. (eds) (2009) *Digital Cityscapes: Merging Digital and Urban Play Spaces*, New York: Peter Lang.

De Souza, E., Silva, A. and Frith, J. (2012) *Mobile Interfaces in Public Spaces: Locational Privacy, Control and Urban Sociability*, New York: Routledge.

De Vogli, R. (2011) 'Neoliberal globalisation and health in a time of economic crisis', *Social Theory & Health*, 9(4): 311–332.

Decew, J.W. (1997) *Pursuit of Privacy: Law, Ethics, and the Rise of Technology*, Ithaca, NY: Cornell University Press.

Deibert, R. and Rohozinski, R. (2010) 'Liberation vs control: the future of cyberspace', *The Journal of Democracy*, 21(4): 43–57.

Deleuze, G. (1992) 'Postscript on the societies of control', *JSTOR*, 59: 3–7.

Dentzer, S. (2013) 'Rx for the "blockbuster drug" of patient engagement', *Health Affairs (Millwood)*, 32(2): 202, doi: 10.1377/hlthaff.2013.0037.

Denzin, N. (1970) *The Research Act in Sociology: A Theoretical Introduction to Sociological Methods*, London: Butterworth.

Department of Health (2011) 'Healthy lives, healthy people: call to action on obesity', Gov.uk, 13 October, Available from: https://www.gov.uk/government/uploads/system/uploads/attachment_data/file/134840/dh_130487.pdf [Accessed 5 October 2015].

Depper, A. and Howe, P.D. (2017) 'Are we fit yet? English adolescent girls' experiences of health and fitness apps', *Health Sociology Review*, 26(1): 98–112.

Dodge, M. and Kitchin, R. (2007) 'Outlines of a world coming into existence: pervasive computing and the ethics of forgetting', *Planning & Design*, 34(3): 431–445.

Dolan, B. (2013) 'Roundup: predictions for digital health in 2013', Mobile Health News, 3 January, Available from: http://mobihealthnews.com/19712/roundup-predictions-for-digital-health-in-2013/ [Accessed 16 October 2015].

Dong, G. and Potenza, M.N. (2014) 'A cognitive-behavioural model of internet gaming disorder: theoretical underpinnings and clinical implications', *Journal of Psychiatric Research*, 58: 7–11.

Dong, G.H., DeVito, E.E., Du, X.X. and Cui, Z.Y. (2012) 'Impaired inhibitory control in "internet addiction disorder": a functional magnetic resonance imaging study', *Psychiatry Research: Neuroimaging*, 203(3): 153–158.

Dosekun, S. (2015) 'For western girls only? Post-feminism as transnational culture', *Feminist Media Studies*, 15(6): 960–975.

Dosekun, S. (2016) 'The risky business of postfeminist beauty', in Elias, A., Gill, R. and Scharff, C. (eds) (2016) *Aesthetic Labour: Rethinking Beauty Politics in Neoliberalism*, Basingstoke: Palgrave Macmillan.

Doyle, A. (2011) 'Revisiting the synopticon: reconsidering Mathiesen's "The Viewer Society" in the age of web 2.0', *Theoretical Criminology*, 15(3): 283–299.

Dubrofsky, R.E. and Magnet, S. (eds) *Feminist Surveillance Studies*, Durham: Duke University Press.

Duffy, D. (2014) 'The digital human. "Quantisize"', BBC Radio 4, 28 April, Available from: https://www.bbc.co.uk/programmes/b041vvw2 [Accessed 1 June 2018].

Dyer, J. (2016) 'Quantified bodies', *Digital Culture & Society*, 2(1): 161–168.

Eco, U. (1976) *A Theory of Semiotics*, Bloomington: Indiana University Press/London: Macmillan.

Elias, A., Gill, R. and Scharff, C. (eds) (2016) *Aesthetic Labour: Rethinking Beauty Politics in Neoliberalism*, Basingstoke: Palgrave Macmillan.

Elias, A.S. and Gill, R. (2017) 'Beauty surveillance: the digital self-monitoring cultures of neoliberalism', *European Journal of Cultural Studies*, 21(1): 59–77.

Elliot, A. and Urry, J. (2010) *Mobile Lives*, Oxford: Routledge.

Ellis, C. (2004) *The Ethnographic I: A Methodological Novel about Autoethnography*, Walnut Creek, CA: AltaMira Press.

Elmer, G. (2003) 'A diagram of panoptic surveillance', *New Media & Society*, 5(2): 231–247.

Enli, G. (2015) *Mediated Authenticity: How the Media Constructs Reality*, New York: Peter Lang.

Entwistle, V.A., Renfrew, M.J., Yearley, S., Forrester, J. and Lamont, T. (1998) 'Lay perspectives: advantages for health research', *British Medical Journal*, 316: 463–466.

Epstein, R. (2004) 'In defence of the old public health: the legal framework for the regulation of public health', *Brooklyn Law Review*, 69: 1421.

Epstein, S. (1994) 'Integration of the cognitive and the psychodynamic unconscious', *American Psychology*, 49(8): 709–724. doi: 10.1037//0003-066x.49.8.709.

Epstein, S. and Timmermans, S. (2021) 'From medicine to health: the proliferation and diversification of cultural authority', *Journal of Health and Social Behavior*, 62(3): 240–254. https://doi.org/10.1177/00221465211010468.

European Commission General Data Protection Regulation (2018) '2018 reform of EU data protection rules', EC.Europa.eu, May, Available from: https://ec.europa.eu/commission/priorities/justice-and-fundamental-rights/data-protection/2018-reform-eu-data-protection-rules_en [Accessed 1 June 2018].

European Commission Green Paper (2014) 'Mobile health', Brussels, 10 April, COM(2014)219 final, Available from: https://ec.europa.eu/digital-single-market/en/news/green-paper-mobile-health-mhealth [Accessed 31 May 2018].

Facebook (2018) 'About', 20 May, Available from: https://www.facebook.com/pg/facebook/about/?ref=page_internal [Accessed 4 June 2018].

Fage-Butler, A. (2018) 'Sleep app discourses: A cultural perspective', in Ajana, B. (ed) *Metric Culture*, Bingley: Emerald Publishing Limited, 157–176.

Fajans, J. (2013) 'Self-experimentation & the quantified self: new avenues for positive psychology research and application', Master's thesis, Claremont Graduate University, California, Available from: https://www.slideshare.net/mrboodaddy/self-experimentation-the-quantified-self-new-avenues-for-positive-psychology-research-and-applicaiton [Accessed 4 May 2017].

Faulkner, K.K. and Duecker, S.J. (1989) 'Stress, time distortion, and failure to recover among obese individuals: implications for weight-gain and dieting', *International Journal of Eating Disorders*, 8(2): 247–250.

Featherstone, M. (1991) *Consumer Culture and Post-modernism*, London: SAGE.

Feldman, Z. and Goodman, M.K. (2021) 'Digital food culture, power and everyday life', *European Journal of Cultural Studies*, 24(6): 1227–1242, https://doi.org/10.1177/13675494211055501

Felton, D. (2014) On Duffy, D. (2014) 'Digital Human. "Quantisize"', BBC Radio 4, 28 April, Available from: https://www.bbc.co.uk/programmes/b041vvw2 [Accessed 1 June 2018].

Festinger, L. (1954) 'A theory of social comparison processes', *Human Relations*, 7(2): 117–140.

Finley, K. (2013) 'What if your boss tracked your sleep, diet, and exercise?', *Wired*, 17 April, Available from: http://www.wired.com/wiredenterprise/2013/04/quantified-work-citizen/ [Accessed 5 May 2018].

Fiske, J. (1987). Television Culture (1st ed.). Routledge. https://doi.org/10.4324/9780203133446

Flinterman, J.F., Teclemariam-Mesbah, R., Broerse, J.E.W. and Bunders, J.F.G. (2001) 'Transdisciplinarity: the new challenge for biomedical research', *Bulletin of Science, Technology & Society*, 21(4): 253–266.

Florida, R. (2002) *The Rise of the Creative Class*, New York: Basic Books.

Foer, J.S. (2013) 'How not to be alone', *New York Times*, Sunday Review, 8 June, Available from: https://www.nytimes.com/2013/06/09/opinion/sunday/how-not-to-be-alone.html [Accessed 14 May 2018].

Forlano, L. (2013) 'Making waves: urban technology and the co-production of place', *First Monday*, 18(4), doi: https://doi.org/10.5210/fm.v18i11.4968.

Forlano, L. (2018) 'Invisible algorithms, invisible politics', *Public Books*, 2 February, Available from: http://www.publicbooks.org/invisible-algorithms-invisible-politics/ [Accessed 2 June 2018].

Fotopoulou, A. (2014) 'The quantified self community, lifelogging and the making of "smart" publics', OpenDemocracy.Net. 10 September, Available from: https://www.opendemocracy.net/participation-now/aristea-fotopoulou/quantified-self-community-lifelogging-and-making-of-%E2%80%9Csmart%E2%80%9D-pub [Accessed 25 May 2018].

Fotopoulou, A. and O'Riordan, K. (2016) 'Training to self-care: fitness tracking, biopedagogy and the healthy consumer', *Health Sociology Review*, 26(1): 54–68.

Foucault, M. (1961/2006) *History of Madness*, London and New York: Routledge.

Foucault, M. (1963/2010) *The Birth of the Clinic: An Archaeology of Medical Perception*, London and New York: Routledge.

Foucault, M. (1966/2002) *The Order of Things: An Archaeology of the Human Sciences*, London and New York: Routledge.

Foucault, M. (1969) *The Archaeology of Knowledge*, Paris: Éditions Gallimard.

Foucault, M. (1971/1977) 'Nietzsche, genealogy, history', in D.F. Bouchard (ed) *Language, Counter-Memory, Practice: Selected Essays and Interviews*, Ithaca: Cornell University Press, 139–164.

Foucault, M. (1974/2000) 'The birth of social medicine', in P. Rabinow (ed) *Michel Foucault, Essential Works III: Power*, New York: The New Press, 134–156.

Foucault, M. (1979a) *Discipline and Punish: The Birth of the Prison*, Harmondsworth: Penguin.

Foucault, M. (1979b) *The Will to Knowledge: The History of Sexuality*, Vol. I, London: Allen Lane.

Foucault, M. (1980) *Power/Knowledge: Selected Interviews and Other Writings 1972–1977* (ed C. Gordon), New York: Pantheon Books.

Foucault, M. (1980a/1996) 'The impossible prison', in S. Lotringer (ed) *Foucault Live: Collected Interviews, 1961–1984*, New York: Semiotext(e), 275–286.

Foucault, M. (1980b/1991) 'Questions of method', in G. Burchell, C. Gordon and P. Miller (eds) *The Foucault Effect: Studies in Governmentality*, Chicago: The University of Chicago Press, 73–86.

Foucault, M. (1986) *The Care of the Self: The History of Sexuality*, Vol. 3, New York: Random House.

Foucault, M. (1988) 'Technologies of the self', in L.H. Martin, H. Gutman and P.H. Hutton (eds) *Technologies of the Self: A Seminar with Michel Foucault*, Amherst: University of Massachusetts Press, 16–49.

Foucault, M. (1990) 'Politics and reason', in L.D. Kritzman (ed) *Michel Foucault, Politics, Philosophy, Culture, Interviews and Other Writings 1977–1984*, New York and London: Routledge, 57–87.

Foucault, M. (1997a) *Essential Works of Foucault, Vol. 1: Ethics: Subjectivity and Truth* (ed P. Rabinow), New York: The New Press.

Foucault, M. (1997b) 'The birth of biopolitics', in M. Foucault (auth) *Ethics: Subjectivity and Truth* (ed P. Rabinow), New York: The New Press. 73–79.

Foucault, M. (1998) *The History of Sexuality*, Vol. 1, London: Penguin.

Foucault, M. (2003) *Society Must Be Defended: Lectures at the Collège de France* 1975–1976, New York: Picador.

Foucault, M. (2007) *Security, Territory, Population: Lectures at the Collège de France*, 1977–78, London: Palgrave Macmillan.

Foucault, M. (2008) *The Birth of Biopolitics: Lectures at the Collège de France*, 1978–9, Basingstoke: Palgrave Macmillan.

Fourcade, M. and Healy, K. (2017) 'Seeing like a market', *Socio-Economic Review*, 15(1): 9–29.

Fox, S. and Duggan, M. (2012) 'Mobile health', Pew Research Centre, Available from: http://www.pewinternet.org/~/media//Files/Reports/2012/PIP_MobileHealth2012.pdf [Accessed 3 June 2015].

Fox, S. and Duggan, M. (2013) 'Tracking for health', Pew Research Centre, Available from: http://www.pewinternet.org/~/media//Files/Reports/2013/PIP_TrackingforHealth_PDF.pd [Accessed 13 June 2021].

Fraisse, P. (1984) 'Perception and estimation of time', *Annual Review of Psychology*, 35(1): 1–36.

Frank, R.H. (1988) *Passions within Reason: The Strategic Role of the Emotions*, New York: Norton.

Freberg, K., Graham, K., McGaughey, K. and Freberg, L. (2010) 'Who are the social media influencers? A study of public perceptions of personality', *Public Relations Review*, 37(1): 90–92.

Frith, E. (2017) 'Social media and children's mental health: a review of the evidence', Education Policy Institute, 30 June, Available from: https://epi.org.uk/publications-and-research/social-media-childrens-mental-health-review-evidence/ [Accessed 25 May 2020].

Fullagar, S. (2008) 'Sites of somatic subjectivity: e-scaped mental health promotion and the bio-politics of depression', *Social Theory & Health*, 6(4): 323–341.

Fuller, M. (ed) (2008) *Software Studies: A Lexicon*, Cambridge, MA: MIT Press.

Gaesser, G. (2002) *Big Fat Lies: The Truth about Your Weight and Your Health*, Carlsbad. Gurze Books.

Gagnon, M., Jacob, J.D. and Holmes, D. (2010) 'Governing through (in) security: a critical analysis of a fear-based public health campaign', *Critical Public Health*, 20(2): 245–256.

Galič, M., Timan, T. and Koops, B. (2016) 'Bentham, Deleuze and beyond: an overview of surveillance theories from the panopticon to participation', *Philosophy & Technology*, 30(1): 9–37.

Gandy, O. (1993) *The Panoptic Sort*, Boulder: Westview Press.

Garcia, A.C, Alecea, I., Standlee, J.B. and Yan, C. (2009) 'Ethnographic approaches to the internet and computer-mediated communication', *Journal of Contemporary Ethnography*, 38: 52–84.

Garcia-Gomez, M. (2017) 'Facebook knows Instagram is toxic for teen girls, company documents show', *Wall Street Journal*. Available from: https://www.wsj.com/articles/facebook-knows-instagram-is-toxic-for-teen-girls-company-documents-show-11631620739?mod=e2tw [Accessed 23 February 2023].

Gardner, P. and Wray, B. (2013) 'From lab to living room: transhumanist imaginaries of consumer brain wave monitors', *Ada: A Journal of Gender, New Media and Technology*, 3: np.

Geertz, C. (1973) *The Interpretation of Cultures*, New York: Basic Books.

Georgakopoulou, A. (2013) 'Small stories and identities analysis as a framework for the study of im/politeness-in-interaction', *Journal of Politeness Research*, 9(1): 55–74.

Georgakopoulou, A. (2014) 'Small stories transposition and social media: a micro-perspective on the "Greek crisis"', *Discourse & Society*, 25(4): 519–539.

Gergen, K. (2002) 'Cell phone technology and the realm of absent presence', in J. Katz and M. Aakhus (eds) *Perpetual Contact: Mobile Communication, Private Talk, Public Performance*, New York: Cambridge University Press, 227–242.

Gerlitz, C. and Helmond, A. (2013) 'The like economy: social buttons and the data-intensive web', *New Media & Society*, 15(8): 1348–1365.

Gerlitz, C. and Lury, C. (2014) 'Social media and self-evaluating assemblages: on numbers, orderings and values', *Distinktion: Scandinavian Journal of Social Theory*, 15(2): 174–188.

Gershon, I. (2010) *Breakup 2.0. Disconnecting over New Media*, Ithaca: Cornell University Press.

Giddens, A. (1991) *Modernity and Self-Identity: Self and Society in the Late Modern Age*, Cambridge: Polity Press.

Gill, R. (2007a) *Gender and the Media*, Cambridge: Polity Press.

Gill, R. (2007b) 'Postfeminist media culture: elements of a sensibility', *European Journal of Cultural Studies*, 10(2): 147–166.

Gill, R. (2017) 'The affective, cultural and psychic life of postfeminism', *European Journal of Cultural Studies*, 20(6): 606–626.

Gill, R. and Scharff, C. (2011) 'Introduction', in R. Gill and C. Scharff (eds) *New Femininities: Postfeminism, Neoliberalism and Subjectivity*, Basingstoke: Palgrave Macmillan, 1–17.

Gill, R. and Orgad, S. (2015) 'The confidence culture', *Australian Feminist Studies*, 30: 324–344.

Gilmore, J. (2015) 'Everywear: the quantified self and wearable fitness technologies', *New Media & Society*, 18(11): 2524–2539.

Gilroy-Ware, M. (2017) *Filling the Void: Emotion, Capitalism and Social Media*, London: Repeater Books.

Giroux, H.A. (2002) 'From "manchild" to "baby boy": race and the politics of self-help', *JAC [Journal of Advanced Composition]*, 22(3): 527–560.

Giroux, H.A. (2004) 'Public pedagogy and the politics of neo-liberalism: making the political more pedagogical', *Policy Futures in Education*, 2: 494–503.

Giroux, H.A. (2014) 'Protesting youth in the age of neoliberal cruelty', Available from: http://www.truth-out.org/news/item/24437-protesting-youth-in-an-age-of-neoliberal-savagery [Accessed 18 June 2015].

Glaser, B.G. and Strauss, A.L. (1967) *The Discovery of Grounded Theory: Strategies for Qualitative Research*, Chicago: Aldin.

Glomb, T., Duffy, M., Bono, J. and Yang, T. (2011) 'Mindfulness at work', *Research in Personnel and Human Resources Management*, 30: 115–157. DOI:10.1108/S0742-7301(2011)0000030005.

Goffman, E. (1959) *The Presentation of Self in Everyday Life*, New York: Anchor Books.

Goffman, E. (1961) *Asylums*, Garden City, NY: Anchor Books.

Goffman, E. (1971) *Relations in Public. Micro Studies of the Public Order*, New York: Basic Books.

Goggin, G. and Hjorth, L. (eds) (2014) *The Routledge Companion to Mobile Media*, New York and Oxford: Routledge.

Goldberg, D.S. (2012) 'Social justice, health inequalities and methodological individualism in US health promotion', *Public Health Ethics*, 5(2): 104–115.

Goodyear, V.A. (2017) 'Social media, apps, and wearable technologies: navigating ethical dilemmas and procedures', *Qualitative Research in Sport, Exercise and Health*, 9(3): 285–302.

Goodyear, V.A., Kerner, C. and Quennerstedt, M. (2017) 'Young people's uses of wearable healthy lifestyle technologies: surveillance, self-surveillance and resistance', *Sport, Education and Society*: 24(1) 97–112.

Gordon, E. and da Silva, A. (2011) *Net Locality: Why Location Matters in a Networked World*, Chichester: Wiley-Blackwell.

Gray, A. (2003) *Research Practices for Cultural Studies*, London: SAGE.

Gray, M.A. (1982) 'Inequalities in health. The Black Report: a summary and comment', *International Journal of Health Services*, 12(3): 349 – 380.

Greene, J. and Hubbard, J.H. (2012) 'Why does patient activation matter? An examination of the relationships between patient activation and health-related outcomes', *Journal of General Internal Medicine*, 27(5): 520–526.

Greenfield, A. (2006) *Everyware: The Dawning Age of Ubiquitous Computing*, Berkeley: New Riders.

Greenfield, L. (2016) 'Deep data: notes on the n of 1', in D. Nafus (ed) *Quantified: Bio-sensing Technologies in Everyday Life*, Cambridge, MA: MIT Press, 123–124.

Gregg, M. (2011) *Work's Intimacy*, Cambridge: Polity Press.

Gregory, A. (2013) 'Is our tech obsession making anorexia worse?', *The New Republic*, 18 December, Available from: http://www.newrepublic.com/article/115969/smartphones-and-weight-loss-how-apps-can-make-eating-disorders-worse [Accessed 25 May 2018].

Groening, S. (2010) 'From "a box in the theater of the world" to "the world as your living room": cellular phones, television, and mobile privatisation', *New Media & Society*, 12(8): 1331–1347.

Guyard, C. and Kaun, A. (2018) 'Workfulness: governing the disobedient brain', *Journal of Cultural Economy*, 11(6): 535–548.

Haggerty, K. and Ericson, R. (2006) 'The surveillant assemblage', *British Journal of Sociology*, 51(4): 605–622.

Haggerty, K. and Samatas, M. (2010) *Surveillance and Democracy*, London: Routledge.

Hall, S. (1980) 'Encoding and decoding', in S. Hall, D. Hobson, A. Lowe and P. Willis (eds) *Culture, Media, Language*, London: Hutchinson, 128–138.

Hall, S. (1997) *Representation: Cultural Representations and Signifying Practices*, London: SAGE.

Hall, S. (1999) *Visual Culture: The Reader*, London: SAGE.

Haraway, D. (1991) *Simians, Cyborgs and Women: The Reinvention of Nature*, London: Free Association.

Hardt, M. and Negri, A. (2001) *Empire*, Cambridge: Cambridge University Press.

Harrison, R., Newholm, T. and Shaw, D. (2005) *The Ethical Consumer*, London: SAGE.

Harvey, D. (2005) *A Brief History of Neoliberalism*, New York: Oxford University Press.

Haussmann, J.D., Touloumtzis, C., White, M.T., Colbert, M.D. and Golding, H.C. (2017) 'Adolescent and young adult use of social media for health and its implications', *Journal of Adolescent Health*, 60(6): 714–719.

Hayward, M. (2013) 'ATMs, teleprompters and photo booths: a short history of neoliberal optics', *New Formations*, 80–81: 194–208.

He, Q., Turel, O. and Bechara, A. (2017a) 'Brain anatomy alterations associated with Social Networking Site (SNS) addiction', *Science Reports*, 7(article 45064): 1–8. https://doi.org/10.1038/srep45064.

He, Q., Turel, O., Brevers, D. and Bechara, A. (2017b) 'Excess social media use in normal populations is associated with amygdala-striatal but not with prefrontal morphology', *Psychiatry Research Neuroimaging*, 269(1): 31–35.

Hearn, A. (2008) '"Meat, mask, burden": probing the contours of the branded "self"', *Journal of Consumer Culture*, 8(2): 197–217.

Henry, J. (1948) 'Common problems of research in anthropology and psychiatry', *American Journal of Orthopsychiatry*, XVIII: 698–703.

Herring, S.C. (2004) 'Computer-mediated discourse analysis: an approach to researching online behaviour', in S. Barab, R. Kling and J. Gray (eds) *Designing for Virtual Communities in the Service of Learning*, New York: Cambridge University Press, 338–376.

Hesmondhalgh, D. (2007) *The Cultural Industries*, London: SAGE.

Heussner, K.M. (2013) 'It's not just about big data: here's why small data matters to your health', 17 April, Available from: http://gigaom.com/2013/04/17/its-not-just-about-big-data-heres-why-small-data-matters-to-your-health/ [Accessed 25 May 2018].

Hey, V. (2005) 'The contrasting social logics of sociality and survival: cultures of classed be/longing in late modernity', *Sociology*, 39(5): 855–872.

Heyes, C.J. (2006) 'Foucault goes to weight watchers', *Hypatia*, 21: 126–149.

Hinchcliffe, S. and Woodward, K. (2004) *The Natural and the Social: Uncertainty, Risk, and Change*, London: Routledge.

Hine, C. (2000) *Virtual Ethnography*, London: SAGE.

Hine, C. (2013[2005]) 'Virtual methods and the sociology of cyber-social-scientific knowledge', in C. Hine (ed) *Virtual Methods: Issues in Social Research on the Internet*, London: Bloomsbury, 1–13.

Hjorth, L. (2011) 'Mobile@game cultures: the place of urban mobile gaming', *Convergence*, 17(4): 357–371.

Hogan, B. (2010) 'The presentation of self in the age of social media: distinguishing performances and exhibitions online', *Bulletin of Science, Technology & Society*, 30(6): 377–386.

Holmberg, C., Bischof, C. and Bauer, S. (2012) 'Making predictions: computing populations', *Science, Technology & Human Values*, 38(3): 398–420.

Holmberg, C., Chaplin, E.J., Hillman, T. and Berg, C. (2016) 'Adolescents' presentations of food in social media: an explorative study', *Appetite*, 99: 121–129.

Hook, D. (2007) *Foucault, Psychology and the Analytics of Power*, Basingstoke: Palgrave Macmillan.

Hookway, N. (2017) 'The moral class, narcissism and the problem of do-it-yourself moralities', *The Sociological Review*, 66(1): 107–121.

Hookway, N. and Graham, T. (2017) '"22 push-ups for a cause": depicting the moral self via social media campaign #Mission22', *Journal of Media and Culture*, 20(4), Available from: http://journal.media-culture.org.au/index.php/mcjournal/article/view/1270 [Accessed 30 May 2018].

Hoskins, T. (2014) *Stitched Up: The Anti-capitalist Book of Fashion*, London: Pluto, Available from: http://www.publicbooks.org/invisible-algorithms-invisible-politics/ [Accessed 25 May 2018].

Humphreys, L. and Liao, T. (2013) 'Foursquare and the parochialisation of public space', *First Monday*, 18(11), doi: https://doi.org/10.5210/fm.v18i11.4966.

Husain, I. and Spence, D. (2015) 'Can healthy people benefit from health apps?', *British Medical Journal*, 350, doi: 10.1136/bmj.h1887.

Hymes, D. (1996) *Ethnography, Linguistics, Narrative Inequality. Towards an Understanding of Voice*, London: Taylor & Francis.

Idhe, D. (1999) *Technology and the Lifeworld: From Garden to Earth*, Bloomington and Indianapolis: Indiana University Press.

Instagram (2018) 'About us', 20 May, Available from: https://www.instagram.com/about/us/ [Accessed 4 June 2020].

Jakala, A. and Berki, E. (2004) 'Exploring the principles of individual and group identity in virtual communities', *IADIS International Conference Web Based Communities*, 19–26, Available from: https://www.researchgate.net/publication/267794585_EXPLORING_THE_PRINCIPLES_OF_INDIVIDUAL_AND_GROUP_IDENTITY_IN_VIRTUAL_COMMUNITIES [Accessed 4 May 2021].

James, C. (2014) *Disconnected: Youth, New Media and the Ethics Gap*, London: MIT Press.

Jenkins, H. (2006) *Convergence Culture: Where Old and New Media Collide*, New York: New York University Press.

Jespersen, J.L., Albrechtslund, A., Øhrstrøm, P., Hasle, P.F.V. and Albretsen, J. (2007) 'Surveillance, Persuasion, and Panopticon', in Y. de Kort, W. IJsselsteijn, C. Midden, B. Eggen and B.J. Fogg (eds) Persuasive Technology: Second International Conference on Persuasive Technology, PERSUASIVE 2007: Revised Selected Papers. IEEE Computer Society Press, Lecture Notes in Computer Science, vol. 4744/2007, 109–120, International Conference on Persuasive Technology, PERSUASIVE 2007, Palo Alto, United States, 26 April.

Johnson, E., Shu, S., Dellaert, B., Fox, C., Goldstein, D., Haubl, G., Larrick, R., Payne, J., Peters, E., Schkade, D. Wansink, B. and Weber, E. (2012) 'Beyond nudges: tools of a choice architecture', *Marketing Letters*, 23(2): 487–504.

Kaneshige, T. (2012) 'The 10 best iPhone apps for healthy living', *CIO*, 4 January, Available from: http://www.cio.com/article/2368089/apple-phone/10-best-iphone-apps-for-healthy-living.html#slide1 [Accessed 16 October 2015].

Kaplan, R.M. and Stone, A.A. (2013) 'Bringing the laboratory and clinic to the community: mobile technologies for health promotion and disease prevention', *Annual Review of Psychology*, 64(1): 471–498.

Karl, I. (2009) 'Technology and women's lives: queering media ethnography', *Reconstruction*, Special Issue on Fieldwork and Interdisciplinary Research, 9(1): np.

Katz, J. and Aakhus, M. (2002) *Perpetual Contact: Mobile Communication, Private Talk, Public Performance*, New York: Cambridge University Press.

Kawachi, I. (2002) 'Social epidemiology', *Social Science and Medicine*, 54(12): 1739–1741.

Keen, A. (2015) *The Internet Is Not the Answer*, London: Atlantic.

Kelly, K. (2011) 'Self-Tracking? You Will', *The Technium*, 25 March, Available from: http://www.kk.org/thetechnium/archives/2011/03/self-tracking_y.php [Accessed 13 June 2015].

Kelly, K. and Wolf, G. (2007) 'Lifelogging, an inevitability', *The Technium*, 20 October, Available from: www.kk.org/thetechnicum:http://www.kk.org/thetechnium/archives/2007/02/lifelogging_an.php [Accessed 13 June 2015].

Kelly, K. and Wolf, G. (2010) 'The quantified century', Quantified Self Conference, Stanford University, Palo Alto, CA, 15–16 September, Available from: http://quantifiedself .com/conference/Palo-Alto-2012 [Accessed 1 May 2015].

Kelly, K., Wolf, G., Carmichael, A. and Ramirez, E. (eds) (2007) 'Quantified self about', Available from: http://www.kk.org/thetechnium/archives/2011/03/self-tracking_y.php [Accessed 13 June 2015].

Kelvin, P. (1973) 'A social-psychological examination of privacy', *British Journal of Clinical Psychology*, 12(3): 248–261.

Kent, R. (2018) 'Social media and self-tracking: representing the "health self"', in B. Ajana (ed) *Self-Tracking: Empirical and Philosophical Investigations*, Cham: Palgrave Macmillan, 61–76.

Kent, R. (2020a) 'COVID-19, toxic productivity & technology overload: our new visceral digital life', *Metric Life*, November, Available from: https://metriclife.net/publications/covid-19-toxic-productivity-technology-overload-our-new-visceral-digital-life/ [Accessed 29 April 2021].

Kent, R. (2020b) 'Should we all social media detox after the pandemic', *Forbes*, Commentary, 7 May.

Kent, R. (2020c) 'Self-tracking and digital food cultures: surveillance and representation of the moral "healthy" body', in D. Lupton and Z. Feldman (eds) *Digital Food Cultures*, Abingdon: Routledge, 19–34.

Kent, R. (2020d) 'Self-tracking health over time: from the use of Instagram to perform optimal health to the protective shield of the digital detox', *Social Media +Society Special Issue: Studying Instagram Beyond Selfies*, 6(3): 1–14.

Kent, R. (2021) 'Digital food tracking: combining traditional and digital ethnographic methods to identify the influence of social media sharing of health and food upon users' everyday lives', in S. Krogager, G. Stinne and J. Leer (eds) *Research Methods in Digital Food Studies*, New York: Routledge., 143–163.

Kent, R. (2022a) 'From the welfare state to digital self-care: historical context of tracking health and quantifying bodies', in B. Ajana (ed) *The Quantification of Bodies in Health*, Bingley: Emerald, 71–92.

Kenten, C. (2010) 'Narrating oneself: reflections on the use of solicited diaries with diary interviews', *Forum: Qualitative Social Research*, 11(2): np.

King, M. and Watson, K. (2005) *Representing Health: Discourses of Health and Illness in the Media*, Basingstoke: Palgrave Macmillan.

Kirkpatrick, R. (2013) 'A new type of philanthropy: Donating data', Available from: https://hbr.org/2013/03/a-new-type-of-philan-thropy-don&cm_sp=Article-_-Links-_-Top%20of%20Page%20Recirculation [Accessed 1 February 2016].

Kitchin, R. and Dodge, M. (eds) (2011) *Code/Space Software and Everyday Life*, Cambridge, MA: MIT Press.

Kleinman, A. (2018) Interview with Karen Barad 'Intra-Actions'. Available from: https://www.academia.edu/1857617/_Intra_actions_Interview_of_Karen_Barad_by_Adam_Kleinmann_

Knowles, P. (1997) 'Moralisation', in M. Brandt and P. Rozin (eds) *Morality and Health*, London: Routledge, 379–401.

Korda, H. and Itani, Z. (2013) 'Harnessing social media for health promotion and behaviour change', *Health Promotion Practice*, 14(1): 15–23.

Kosinski, M., Stillwell, D. and Graepel, T. (2013) 'Private traits and attributes are predictable from digital records of human behaviour', *Proceedings of the National Academy of Sciences*, 10(15): 5802–5805.

Kozinets, R.V. (2009) *Netnography: Doing Ethnographic Research Online*, London: SAGE.

Krieger, N. (2001) 'A glossary for social epidemiology', *Journal of Epidemiology and Community Health*, 55(10): 693–700.

Krieger, N. (2007) 'Why epidemiologists cannot afford to ignore poverty', *Epidemiology*, 18(6): 658–663.

Kristensen, D.B. and Prigge, C. (2018) 'Human/technology associations in self-tracking practices', in B. Ajana (ed) *Self-Tracking: Empirical and Philosophical Investigations*, Cham: Palgrave Macmillan, 43–60.

Kristensen, D.B. and Ruckenstein, M. (2018) 'Co-evolving with self-tracking technologies', *New Media & Society*, 5(3): 219–238.

Kristensen, D.B., Lim, M. and Askegaard, S. (2016) 'Healthism in Denmark: state, market, and the search for a "moral compass"', *Health*, 20(5): 485–504.

Lair, D., Sullivan, K. and Cheney, G. (2015) 'Marketization and the recasting of the professional self: the rhetoric and ethics of personal branding', *Management Communication Quarterly*, 18(3): 307–343.

Lang, T., Barling, D. and Caraher, M. (2004) 'Food policy: integrating health environment, and society', Oxford Scholarship Online, Available from: https://oxford.universitypressscholarship.com/view/10.1093/acprof:oso/9780198567882.001.0001/acprof-9780198567882-indexList-1 [Accessed 29 April 2020].

Langwieser, C. and Kirig, A. (2010) *Konsument 2020*, Kelkheim: Zukunftsinstitut.

Lansley, A. (2008) 'No excuses, no nannying', Conservatives.com, 27 August, Available from: http://www.conservatives.com/News/Speeches/2008/08/Andrew_Lansley_No_excuses_no_nannying.aspx [Accessed 4 January 2015].

Latour, B. (1992) 'Where are the missing masses? The sociology of a few mundane artifacts', in W. E. Bijker and J. Law (eds) *Shaping Technology/Building Society: Studies in Sociotechnical Change*, Cambridge, MA: MIT Press, 225–258.

Lavers, A. (1982) *Roland Barthes: Structuralism and After*, London: Methuen.

Lawrence, B. (2004) 'Framing obesity: the evolution of news discourse on a public health issue', *Press/Politics*, 9(3): 56–75.

Lazar, A., Koehler, C. and Tanenbaum, J. (2015) 'Why we use and abandon smart devices', Proceedings of the 2015 ACM international joint conference on pervasive and ubiquitous computing, Osaka, Japan, 7–11 September, New York: ACM, 635–646.

Lazzarato, M. (2006) '"Semiotic pluralism" and the new government of signs – homage to Félix Guattari', EIPCP, Available from: http://eipcp.net/transversal/0107/lazzarato/en [Accessed 25 May 2021].

Leahy, D., Burrows, L., McCuaig, L., Wright, J. and Penney, D. (2016) *School Health Education in Changing Times*, London: Routledge.

LeBesco, K. (2011) 'Neoliberalism, public health, and the moral perils of fatness', *Critical Public Health*, 21(2): 153–164.

Lederer, A.M., Hoban, M.T., Lipson, S.K., Zhou, S. and Eisenberg, D. (2021) 'More than inconvenienced: the unique needs of U.S. college students during the COVID-19 pandemic', *Health Education & Behavior*, 48(1): 14–19. doi:10.1177/1090198120969372.

Leichter, H. (1997) 'Lifestyle correctness and the new secular morality', in A.M. Brandt and P. Rozin (eds) *Morality and Health*, London: Routledge, 359–378.

Leigh-Hunt, N. et al (2017) 'An overview of systematic reviews on the public health consequences of social isolation and loneliness', *Public Health*, 152: 157–171, doi: 10.1016/j.puhe.2017.07.035.

Leppänen, S., Kytölä, S., Jousmäki, H., Peuronen, S. and Westinen, E. (2013) 'Entextualization and resemiotization as resources for (dis)identification in social media', Tilburg Papers in Culture Studies, Paper 57, Available from: https://www.tilburguniversity.edu/upload/a3d5524e-4413–4772–9f96- 9fe0ee714c6f_TPCS_57_Leppanen-etal.pdf [Accessed 1 May 2018].

Leriche, R. and Arnulf, G. (1936) 'Treatment of sprains by interligamentary injection of novocaine', *The American Journal of Surgery*, 32(1) 45–47. https://doi.org/10.1016/S0002-9610(36)90052-1.

Lesser, L.I., Azar, K.M., Laing, B.Y., Stephens, J., Aurora, M.S., Burke, L.E. and Palaniappan, L.P. (2013) 'Mobile applications for weight management: theory-based content analysis', *American Journal of Preventive Medicine*, 45(5): 583–589.

Lewis, T. (2008) *Smart Living: Lifestyle Media and Popular Expertise*, New York: Peter Lang.

Lianos, M. (2003) 'Social control after Foucault', *Surveillance & Society*, 1(3): 412–430.

Lin, Y.H. et al (2015) 'Time distortion associated with smartphone addiction: identifying smartphone addiction via a mobile application (app)', *Journal of Psychiatric Research*, 65: 139–145.

Lincoln, S. and Robards, B. (2017) 'Editing the project of the self: sustained Facebook use and growing up online', *Journal of Youth Studies*, 20(4): 518–531.

Livingstone, S. (2008) 'Taking risky opportunities in youthful content creation: teenagers' use of social networking sites for intimacy, privacy and self-expression', *New Media & Society*, 10(3): 393–411.

Livingstone, S., Mascheroni, G. and Staksrud, E. (2018) 'European research on children's internet use: Assessing the past and anticipating the future', New Media & Society, 20(3): 1103–1122. https://doi.org/10.1177/1461444816685930.

Lomborg, S. (2011) 'Social media as communicative genres', *Journal of Media and Communication Research*, 51: 55–71.

Lomborg, S. and Frandsen, K. (2016) 'Self-tracking as communication', *Information, Communication & Society*, 19(7): 1015–1027.

Lorig, R. and Holman, M. (2003) 'Self-management education: history, definition, outcomes, and mechanisms', *Annals of Behavioural Medicine*, 26(1): 1–7.

Lortie, C.L. and Guitton, M.J. (2013) 'Internet addiction assessment tools: dimensional structure and methodological status', *Addiction*, 108(7): 1207–1216.

Lucivero, F. and Tamburrini, G. (2007) 'Ethical monitoring of brain-machine interfaces', *AI & Society*, 22(3): 449–460.

Lucivero, F. and Prainsack, B. (2015) 'The lifestylisation of healthcare? "Consumer genomics" and mobile health as technologies for healthy lifestyle', *Applied and Translational Genomics*, 4: 44–49.

Lupton, D. (1995) *The Imperative of Health: Public Health and the Regulated Body*, London: SAGE.

Lupton, D. (1997) 'Foucault and the medicalisation critique', in A. Petersen and R. Bunton (eds) *Foucault, Health and Medicine*, London: Routledge, 94–110.

Lupton, D. (1999) 'Developing the "whole me": citizenship, neo-liberalism and the contemporary health and physical education curriculum', *Critical Public Health*, 9(4): 287–300.

Lupton, D. (2010) 'The new mobile digital technologies, health and the body', *This Sociological Life* – A Blog by Deborah Lupton, Word Press, Available from: http://simplysociology.wordpress.com/2012/06/20/the-new-mobile-digital-technologies-health-and-the-body/ [Accessed 16 October 2015].

Lupton, D. (2012a) *Fat*, London: Routledge.

Lupton, D. (2012) 'M-health and health promotion: the digital cyborg and surveillance society', *Social Theory and Health* 10(3): 229–244.

Lupton, D. (2012c) *Medicine as Culture: Illness, Disease and the Body* (3rd edn), London: SAGE.

Lupton, D. (2012d) 'The quantitative self movement: some sociological perspectives', *This Sociological Life* – A Blog by Deborah Lupton, Word Press, 4 November, Available from: http://simplysociology.wordpress.com/2012/11/04/the-quantitative-self-movement-some-sociological-perspectives/ [Accessed 16 October 2015].

Lupton, D. (2013a) 'The commodification of patient opinion: the digital patient experience economy in the age of big data', *Sydney Health & Society Group Working Papers*, (3), Available from: http://hdl.handle.net/2123/9063 [Accessed 6 October 2014].

Lupton, D. (2013b) 'The digital cyborg assemblage: Haraway's cyborg theory and the new digital health technologies', Preprint, Available from: http://www.academia.edu/3563155/The_digital_cyborg_assemblage_Haraways_cyborg [Accessed 5 October 2015].

Lupton, D. (2013c) 'The digitally engaged patient: self-monitoring and self-care in the digital health era', *Social Theory and Health*, 11: 256–270.

Lupton, D. (2013d) 'Living the quantified self: the realities of self-tracking for health', 11 January, Available from: http://simplysociology.wordpress.com/2013/01/11/living-the-quantified-self-the-realities-of-self-tracking-for-health/ [Accessed 05 October 2015].

Lupton, D. (2013e) 'Quantifying the body: monitoring, performing and configuring health in the age of mHealth technologies', *Critical Public Health*, 23(4): 393–403.

Lupton, D. (2013f) *Self-Tracking, Health and Medicine: Sociological Perspectives*, Abingdon: Routledge.

Lupton, D. (2013g) 'Living the quantified self: the realities of self-tracking for health', *This Sociological Life* – A Blog by Deborah Lupton, Word Press, 13 January, Available from: http://simplysociology.wordpress.com/2013/01/11/living-the-quantified-self-the-realities-of-self-tracking-for-health/?blogsub=confirming#blog_subscription-3 [Accessed 16 October 2014].

Lupton, D. (2014a) 'Beyond the quantified self: the reflexive monitoring self', *This Sociological Life* – A Blog by Deborah Lupton, Word Press, Available from: https://papers.ssrn.com/sol3/papers.cfm?abstract_id=2483549 [Accessed 25 May 2018].

Lupton, D. (2014b) 'Self-tracking modes: reflexive self-monitoring and data practices', Paper presented at Imminent Citizenships: Personhood and Identity Politics in the Informatic Age workshop, Australian National University, Canberra, ACT, Australia. 27 August.

Lupton, D. (2014c) 'Health promotion in the digital era: a critical commentary', *Health Promotion International*, 30(1): 174–183.

Lupton, D. (2014d) 'Apps as artefacts: towards a critical perspective on mobile health and medical apps', *Societies*, 4: 606–622.

Lupton, D. (2015) 'Quantified sex: a critical analysis of sexual and reproductive self-tracking using apps', *Culture, Health & Sexuality*, 17(4): 440–453.

Lupton, D. (2016a) *The Quantified Self*, Cambridge: Polity Press.

Lupton, D. (2016b) 'The diverse domains of quantified selves: self-tracking modes and dataveillance', *Economy and Society*, 45(1): 101–122.

Lupton, D. (2019) '"It's made me a lot more aware": a new materialist analysis of health self-tracking', *Media International Australia*, 171(1): 66–79. https://doi.org/10.1177/1329878X19844042.

Lupton, D. (2020) 'The internet of things: social dimensions', *Sociology Compass*, 14(4): https://doi.org/10.1111/soc4.12770.

Lyon, D. (2001) *Surveillance and Society: Monitoring Everyday Life*, Buckingham and Philadelphia: Open University Press.

Lyon, D. (2003) *Surveillance as Social Sorting: Privacy, Risk and Digital Discrimination*, London: Routledge.

Lyon, D. (2007a) *Consuming Life*, Cambridge: Polity Press.

Lyon, D. (2007b) *Surveillance Studies: An Overview*, Cambridge: Polity Press.

Lyon, D. (2010) 'Surveillance, power and everyday life', in P. Kalantzis-Cope and K. Gherab- Martin (eds) *Emerging Digital Spaces in Contemporary Society*, Basingstoke: Palgrave Macmillan, 107–120.

Lyon, D. and Baumen, Z. (2013) *Liquid Surveillance*, Cambridge: Polity Press.

Lyon, D., Ball, K. and Haggerty, K. (eds) (2012) *International Handbook of Surveillance Studies*, London: Routledge.

Mackay, H. (2005) 'New connections, familiar settings: issues in the ethnographic study of new media use at home', in H. Christine (ed) *Virtual Methods – Issues in Social Research on the Internet*, New York: Macmillan. p.129–140

Magnet, S. (2011) *When Biometrics Fail: Gender, Race, and the Technology of Identity*, Durham: Duke University Press.

Maisonneuve, N., Stevens, M. and Ochab, B. (2010) 'Participatory noise pollution monitoring using mobile phones', *Information Polity: The International Journal of Government & Democracy in the Information Age*, 15(1/2): 51–71.

Mann, S. (1994) *Mediated Reality. MIT Media Lab Technical Report 260*, Cambridge, MA: MIT Press.

Mann, S. (2005) 'Sousveillance and cyborglogs: a 30-year empirical voyage through ethical, legal, and policy issues', *Presence: Teleoperators and Virtual Environments*, 14(6): 625–646.

Mann, S. (2013) 'Veillance and reciprocal transparency: surveillance versus sousveillance, AR glass, lifeglogging, and wearable computing', Available from: https://ieeexplore.ieee.org/document/6613094/ [Accessed 9 May 2018].

Manovich, L. (1989) *Logistics of Perception*, London: Verso.

Manovich, L. (2016) 'Instagram and The Contemporary Image'. Available from: http://manovich.net/content/04-projects/161-instagram-and-contemporary-image/instagram_book_manovich_2017.pdf [Accessed 22 February 2023].

Marche, S. (2012) 'Is Facebook making us lonely?', *The Atlantic*, May, Available from: https://www.theatlantic.com/magazine/archive/2012/05/is-facebook-making-us-lonely/308930/ [Accessed 31 May 2018].

Mardawi, A. (2013) 'Your body isn't a temple, it's a data factory emitting digital exhaust', *The Guardian*, Available from: https://www.theguardian.com/commentisfree/2013/jan/25/body-data-factory-digital-exhaust-data-tax [Accessed 25 May 2020].

Marteau, T.M, Ogilvie, D., Roland, M., Suhrcke, M. and Kelly, M.P. (2011) 'Judging nudging: can nudging improve population health?', *BMJ*, 342:d228, doi:10.1136/bmj.d228.

Martinez-Martin, N., Dasgupta, I., Carter, A,, Chandler, J.A., Kellmeyer, P., Kreitmair, K., Weiss, A. and Cabrera, L.Y. (2020) 'Ethics of digital mental health during COVID-19: crisis and opportunities', *JMIR Mental Health*, 7(12): e23776. doi: 10.2196/23776.

Marwick, A.E. and boyd, d. (2010) 'I tweet honestly, I tweet passionately: Twitter users, context collapse, and the imagined audience', *New Media & Society*, 13(1): 114–133.

Marx, G.T. (1985) 'The surveillance society: the threat of 1984-style techniques', *The Futurist*, 6: 21–26.

Marx, G.T. (2001) 'Murky conceptual waters: the public and the private', *Ethics and Information Technology*, 3(3): 157–169.

Maslow, A.H. (1987) *Motivation and Personality* (3rd edn), New York: Harper.

Mason, J. (2002) *Qualitative Researching*, London: SAGE.

Mathes, B.M., Norr, A.M., Allan, N.P., Albanese, B.J. and Schmidt, N.B. (2018) 'Cyberchondria: Overlap with health anxiety and unique relations with impairment, quality of life, and service utilization', *Psychiatry Research*, 261: 204–211. doi: 10.1016/j.psychres.2018.01.002.

Mathiesen, T. (1997) 'The viewer society: Michel Foucault's "panopticon" revisited', *Theoretical Criminology*, 1(2): 215–234.

Mayor-Schönberger, V. and Cukier, K. (2013b) 'Big data: a revolution that will transform how we live, work and think', Available from: https://psycnet.apa.org/record/2013-17650-000 [Accessed 29 April 2021].

McGuigan, J. (2012) 'The coolness of capitalism today', *TripleC*, 10(2): 425–438.

McNair, B. (2003) *An Introduction to Political Communication*, London: Routledge.

McRobbie, A. (2009) *The Aftermath of Feminism: Gender, Culture and Social Change*, London: SAGE.

McRobbie, A. (2015) 'Notes on the perfect: competitive femininity in neoliberal times', *Australian Feminist Studies*, 30(83): 3–20.

Meijer, R. Rijshouwer, Y. and Linse, I. (1993) *Voorlichtuin vanuit het patientenperspectief: een handleiding voor patientenorganisaties* [Information from the patient's perspective: A guide for patients' organisations], Utrecht: Nederlandse Patienten/Consumenten Federatie.

Mello, M.M. and Rosenthal, M.B. (2008) 'Wellness programs and lifestyle discrimination — the legal limits', *The New England Journal of Medicine*, 359(2): 192–199.

Mennel, S. Murcott, A. and van Otterloo, A. (1992) *The Sociology of Food: Eating, Diet and Culture*, London: SAGE.

Mental Health Foundation (2020). 'Body image report', Available at: https://www.mentalhealth.org.uk/explore-mental-health/articles/body-image-report-executive-summary [Accessed 23 February 2023].

Merson, F. and Perriot, J. (2011) 'Social deprivation and time perception, the impact on smoking cessation', *Sante Publique*, 23(5): 359–370.

Mertens, D.M. (1998) *Research Methods in Education and Psychology: Integrating Diversity with Quantitative and Qualitative Approaches*, Thousand Oaks, CA: Sage.

Meth, P. (2003) 'Entries and omissions: using solicited diaries in geographical research', *Area*, 35: 195–205.

Metzl, J. and Kirkland, A. (2010) *Against Health: How Health became the New Morality*, New York: NYU Press.

Meyrowitz, J. (1986) *No Sense of Place: The Impact of Electronic Media on Social Behavior*. New York: Oxford University Press.

Mindell, J., Erens, B., Nelson, M. and Finglas, P. (2007) 'The low income diet and nutrition survey (LIDNS)', *Food Standards Agency*, 17 August, Available from: https://www.ucl.ac.uk/hssrg/studies/low-income [Accessed 1 June 2018].

Mol, A. (2002) *The Body Multiple: Ontology in Medical Practice*, Durham, NC: Duke University Press.

Mol, A. (2009) 'Living with diabetes: care beyond choice and control', *Lancet*, 373(9677): 1756–1757.

Mol, A. and Law, J. (2004) 'Embodied action, enacted bodies: the example of hypoglycaemia', *Body & Society*, 10: 43–62.

Monaghan, P. (2006) 'Watching the watchers', *Chronicle of Higher Education*, 52(28): 1, 18–25.

Moore, N. (1983) *How to Do Research*, London: Library Association.

Moore, P. (2017) *The Quantified Self in Precarity: Work, Technology and What Counts*, Advances in Sociology series, Abingdon: Routledge.

Moore, P. and Robinson, A. (2016) 'The quantified self: what counts in the neoliberal workplace', *New Media* & Society, 18(11): 2774–2792.

Moore, P., Piwek, L. and Roper, I. (2018) 'The quantified workplace: a study in self-tracking, agility and change management', in B. Ajana (ed) *Self-Tracking: Empirical and Philosophical Investigations*, Cham: Palgrave Macmillan, 93–110.

Moore, P. and Robinson, A. (2016) 'The quantified self: What counts in the neoliberal workplace', *New Media & Society*, 18(11): 2774–2792.

Moore, P.V. (2017) *The Quantified Self in Precarity: Work, Technology and What Counts*, Abingdon: Routledge.

Moore, S. (1993) *Interpreting Audiences – The Ethnography of Media Consumption*, London: SAGE.

Moriarty, M. (1991) *Roland Barthes*, Stanford, CA: Stanford University Press.

Morley, D. (1980) *The Nationwide Audience*, London: BFI.

Morley, D. (2007) *Media, Modernity and Technology – The Geography of the New*, London: Routledge.

Morozov, E. (2011) *The Net Delusion: The Dark Side of Internet Freedom*, New York: Public Affairs.

Mort, M. and Smith, A. (2009) 'Beyond information: intimate relations in sociotechnical practice', *Sociology*, 43(2): 215–223.

Mort, M., Finch, T. and May, C. (2009) 'Making and unmaking telepatients: identity and governance in new health technologies', *Science, Technology & Human Values*, 34(1): 9–33.

Mort, M., Roberts, C. and Callen, B. (2013) 'Ageing with telecare: care or coercion in austerity?', *Sociology of Health and Illness*, 35(6): 799–812.

Murphy, P.D. and Kraidy, M.M. (eds) (2003) *Global Media Studies – Ethnographic Perspectives*, London: Routledge.

Murthy, D. (2008) 'Digital ethnography: an examination of the use of new technologies for social research', *Sociology*, 42(5): 837–855.

Myrdal, G. (1969) *Objectivity in Social Research*, Middletown, CT: Wesleyan University Press.

Nafus, D. and Sherman, J. (2014) 'This one does not go up to 11: the quantified self movement as an alternative big data practice', *International Journal of Communication*, 8: 1784–1794.

Nakamura, L. (2015) 'Afterword: blaming, shaming and the feminization of social media', in R.E. Dubrofsky and A.M. Shoshana (eds) *Feminist Surveillance Studies*, Durham, NC, and London: Duke University Press, 173–191.

Nathanson E. (2013) *Television and Postfeminist Housekeeping: No Time for Mother*, New York: Routledge.

Neff, G. and Nafus, D. (2016) *Self-Tracking*, Cambridge, MA: MIT Press.

Negroponte, N. (1995) *Being Digital*, New York: Alfred A. Knopf.

Nettleton, S. (2004) 'The emergence of e-scaped medicine?', *Sociology*, 38(4): 661–679.

Nettleton, S. (2013) *The Sociology of Health and Illness Polity*, Polity Press: Cambridge and Malden.

Nettleton, S. and Burrows, R. (2003) 'E-scaped medicine? Information, reflexivity and health', *Critical Social Policy*, 23(2): 165–185.

Nicolini, D. (2007) 'Stretching out and expanding work practices in time and space: the case of telemedicine', *Human Relations*, 60(6): 889–920.

Nissenbaum, H. (1998) 'Protecting privacy in an information age: the problem of privacy in public', *Law and Philosophy*, 17: 559–596.

Nogala, D. (1995) 'The future role of technology in policing', in J.P. Brodeur (ed) *Comparisons in Policing: An International Perspective*, Avebury: Aldershot, 191–210.

Noji, E., Kappler, K. and Vormbusch, U. (2021) 'Situating conventions of health: transformations, inaccuracies, and the limits of measuring in the field of self-tracking', *Historical Social Research / Historische Sozialforschung*, 46: 261–284.

Norris, C. and Armstrong, G. (1999) *The Maximum Surveillance Society: The Rise of CCTV*, New York: Oxford University Press.

Novas, C. (2006) 'The political economy of hope: patients' organizations, science and biovalue', *BioSocieties*, 1(3): 289–305.

Ohly, H. et al (2016) 'Attention restoration theory: a systematic review of the attention restoration potential of exposure to natural environments', *Journal of Toxicology and Environmental Health. Part B, Critical Reviews*, 19(7): 305–343, doi: 10.1080/10937404.2016.1196155.

Olson, P. and Tilley, A. (2014) 'The quantified other: Nest and Fitbit chase a lucrative side business', *Forbes*, 4 October, Available from: http://www.forbes.com/sites/parmyolson/2014/04/17/thequantified-other-nest-and-Fitbit-chase-a-lucrative-sidebusiness/ [Accessed 25 May 2018].

Ong, A. (2006) *Neoliberalism as Exception: Mutations in Citizenship and Sovereignty*, Durham, NC: Duke University Press.

O'Shaughnessy, E. (1999) 'Relating to the superego', *International Journal of Psychoanalysis*, 80(5): 861–870. Reprinted in C. Mawson (ed) *Bion Today*, East Sussex: Routledge.

Oswald, M. and Grace, J. (2020) 'The COVID-19 contact tracing app in England and "Experimental Proportionality"', 24 June, *Public Law*, Available at SSRN: https://ssrn.com/abstract=3632870 or http://dx.doi.org/10.2139/ssrn.3632870 [Accessed 23 February 2023].

Oudshoorn, N. (2011) *Telecare Technologies and the Transformation of Healthcare*, Basingstoke: Palgrave Macmillan.

Panksepp, J. (2005) 'On the embodied neural nature of core emotional affects', *Journal of Consciousness Studies*, 12(8–10): 158–184.

Pantzar, M. and Ruckenstein, M. (2017) 'Living the metrics: self-tracking and situated objectivity', *Digital Health*, 3: 1–10.

Papacharissi, Z. (2009) 'The virtual geographies of social networks: a comparative analysis of Facebook, LinkedIn and ASmallWorld', *New Media & Society*, 11(1–2): 199–220.

Papacharissi, Z. (2011) *A Networked Self: Identity, Community and Culture on Social Network Sites*, London: Routledge.

Papacharissi, Z. (2012) 'Without you, I'm nothing: performances of the self on Twitter', *International Journal of Communication*, 6: 1989–2006.

Parker, I. (1999) *Critical Textwork: An Introduction to Varieties of Discourse and Analysis*, Buckingham: Open University Press.

Parks, M. (2011) 'Social network sites as virtual communities', in Z. Papacharissi (ed) *The Networked Self: Identity, Community and Culture on Social Network Sites*, New York: Routledge, 39–58.

Parliamentary Office of Science & Technology (2005) Post Note, No. 244 'Binge Drinking and Public Health', Parliament UK, Available from: http://www.parliament.uk/business/publications/research/post/publications-by-year/pubs2005/ [Accessed 3 January 2020].

Parmar, A. (2012) 'Are you a cyberchondriac who believes in the power of Dr. Google?', MedCityNews, 5 June, Available from: http://medcitynews.com/2012/06/are-you-a-cyberchondriac-who-believes-in-the-power-of-dr-google/ [Accessed 16 October 2020].

Paterson, M. (2005) *Consumption and Everyday Life*, London: Routledge.

Percey, W. (1972) *The Message in a Bottle*, Toronto: McGraw-Hill.

Perloff, R. (2014) 'Social media effects on young women's body image concerns: theoretical perspectives and an agenda for research', *Feminist Forum Review*, doi: 10.1007/s11199-014-0384-6.

Perscheid, C., Benzler, J., Hermann, C., Janke, M., Moyer, D., Laedtke, T., Adeoye, O., Denecke, K., Kirchner, G., Beermann, S., Schwarz, N., Tom-Aba, D. and Krause, G. (2018) 'Ebola outbreak containment: real-time task and resource coordination with SORMAS', *Frontiers in ICT*, 5, 7.

Peters, M.A. (2001) *Poststructuralism, Marxism, and Neoliberalism: Between Theory and Politics*, Lanham: Rowman & Littlefield.

Petersen, A. and Bunton, R. (eds) (1997) *Foucault, Health and Medicine*, New York: Routledge.

PEW Research Centre (2016) 'Social media update', 11 November, Available from: http://www.pewinternet.org/2016/11/11/social-media-update-2016 [Accessed 1 May 2021].

Pink, S. and Fors, V. (2017) 'Being in a mediated world: self-tracking and the mind-body-environment', *Cultural Geography*, 24: 375–388.

Plaisime, M., Robertson-James, C., Mejia, L., Núñez, A., Wolf, J. and Reels, S. (2020) 'Social media and teens: A needs assessment exploring the potential role of social media in promoting health', *Social Media + Society*, 6(1). https://doi.org/10.1177/2056305119886025.

Plummer, K. (2001) *Documents of Life 2: An Invitation to a Critical Humanism*, London: SAGE.

Pogorelc, D. (2013) 'Are we headed toward the over-quantified self?', MedCityNews, 1 January, Available from: http://medcitynews.com/2013/01/are-we-headed-toward-the-over-quantified-self/ [Accessed 16 October 2015].

Poovey, M. (1998) *A History of the Modern Fact: Problems of Knowledge in the Sciences of Wealth and Society*, Chicago and London: The University of Chicago Press.

Poster, M. (1990) *The Mode of Information: Postculturalism and Social Context*, Chicago: The University of Chicago Press.

Postill, J. and Pink, S. (2012) 'Social media ethnography: the digital researcher in a messy web', *Media International Australia*, 145(1): 123–134.

Powell, D. and Fitzpatrick, K. (2015) '"Getting fit basically just means, like, non-fat": children's lessons in fitness and fatness', *Sport, Education and Society*, 20(4): 463–484.

Prainsack, B. (2011) 'The power of prediction: how personal genomics became a policy challenge', *Austrian Journal of Political Science*, 40: 401–415.

Prainsack, B. (2014) 'Personhood and solidarity: what kind of personalised medicine do we want?', *Personalised Medicine*, 11(7): 651–657.

Prainsack, B. (2015) 'Is personalised medicine different?', *British Journal of Sociology*, 66(1): 28–35.

Prainsack, B. and Buyx, A. (2012) 'Lifestyle related diseases and individual responsibility through the prism of solidarity', *Clinical Ethics*, 7(2): 79–85.

Prainsack, B. and Buyx, A. (2013) 'A solidarity-based approach to the governance of research biobanks', *Medical Law Review*, 21(1): 71–91.

Probyn, E. (1993) *Sexing the Self: Gendered Positions in Cultural Studies*, Oxford: Routledge.

Punch, K. (2014) *Introduction to Social Research: Quantitative & Qualitative Approaches*, London: SAGE.

Purpura, S., Schwanda, V., Williams, K., Stubler, W. and Sengers, P. (2011) *Fit4Life: The Design of a Persuasive Technology Promoting Healthy Behavior and Ideal Weight*, Paper presented at the ACM CHI Conference on Human Factors in Computing Systems, Vancouver, BC, Canada, 7–12 May.

Pybus, J., Cote, M. and Blanke, T. (2015) 'Hacking the social life of big data', *Big Data & Society*: 1–10, *Quantified Self at Outlier Consulting*, 13 April,

Quennerstedt, M., Burrows, L. and Maivorsdotter, N. (2010) 'From teaching young people to be healthy to learning health', *Utbildning och Demokrati*, 19(2): 97–112.

Quigley, M. (2013) 'Nudging for health: on public policy and designing choice architecture', *Medical Law Review*, 21: 588–621.

Rabinow, P. (1996) *Essays on the Anthropology of Reason*, Princeton: Princeton University Press.

Rail, G. and Jette, S. (2015) 'Reflections on biopedagogies and/of public health: on bio-others, rescue missions, and social justice', *Cultural Studies ↔ Critical Methodologies*, 15(5): 327–336.

Rail, G. and Lafrance, M. (2009)'Confessions of the flesh and biopedagogies: discursive constructions of obesity on nip/tuck', *Medical Humanities*, 35: 76–79.

Rainford, P. and Tinkler, J. (2011) 'Designing for nudge effects: how behaviour management can ease public sector problems', LSE Public Policy Group. Innovating through Design in Public Sector Services Seminar series, Available from: http://eprints.lse.ac.uk/37810 [Accessed 2 October 2015].

Raphael, D. (2008) 'Grasping at straws: a recent history of health promotion in Canada', *Critical Public Health*, 18(4): 483–495.

Raphael, D. (2011) 'A discourse analysis of the social determinants of health', *Critical Public Health*, 21(2): 221–236.

Raphael, D. (2013) 'The political economy of health promotion: part 1, national commitments to provision of the prerequisites of health', *Health Promotion International*, 28(1): 95–111.

Rau, P.L.P., Peng, S.Y. and Yang, C.C. (2006) 'Time distortion for expert and novice online game players', *Cyberpsychology, Behavior, and Social Networking*, 9(4): 396–403.

Rawassizadeh, R. (2012) 'Towards sharing life-long information with society', *Behaviour & Information Technology*, 31(11): 1057–1067.

Reid, A. (2010) 'Social media, public pedagogy and the end of private learning', in J.A. Sandlin, B.D. Shultz and J. Burdick (eds) *Handbook of Public Pedagogy*, London: Routledge, 194–200.

Rennington, K.A. and Shumar, W. (2002) *Building Virtual Communities: Learning and Changing in Cyberspace*, Cambridge: Cambridge University Press.

Rentzer, S. (2013) 'Rx for the "blockbuster drug" of patient engagement', *Health Affairs*, 32(2): 202.

Rettberg, J.W. (2014) *Seeing Ourselves through Technology: How We Use Selfies, Blogs and Wearable Devices to See and Shape Ourselves*, Basingstoke: Palgrave Macmillan.

Rettberg, J.W. (2018) 'Apps as companions: how quantified self apps become our audience and our companions', in B. Ajana (ed) *Self-Tracking: Empirical and Philosophical Investigations*, Cham: Palgrave Macmillan, 27–42.

Rheingold, H. (2002) *Smart Mobs: The Next Social Revolution*, Cambridge, MA: Perseus.

Rich, E. and Miah, A. (2009) 'Prosthetic surveillance: the medical governance of health bodies in cyberspace', *Surveillance & Society*, 6(2): 163–177.

Rich, E. and Miah, A. (2017) 'Mobile, wearable and ingestible health technologies: towards a critical research agenda', *Health Sociology Review*, 26(1): 84–97.

Ritzer, G. and Jurgenson, N. (2010) 'Production, consumption, prosumption: the nature of capitalism in the age of the digital "prosumer"', *Journal of Consumer Culture*, 10(1): 13–36.

Ritzer, G., Dean, P. and Jurgenson, N. (2012) 'The coming of age of the prosumer', *American Behavioural Scientist*, 56(4): 379–398.

Roach, R. (2017) 'Epilepsy, digital technology and the black-boxed self', *New Media & Society*, 20(8): 1–18. doi: https://doi.org/10.1177/1461444817736926.

Robins, K. and Webster, F. (1999) *Times of the Technoculture: From the Information Society to the Virtual Life*, London: Routledge.

Robinson, L. and Schulz, J. (2009) 'New avenues for sociological inquiry: evolving forms of ethnographic practice', *Sociology*, 43: 685–698.

Rogers, H. (2005) *Writing Systems: A Linguistic Approach*, Malden: Blackwell.

Ronquillo, Y., Meyers, A. and Korvek, S.J. (2020) *Digital Health*, Treasure Island: Statpearls Publishing, Available from: https://pubmed.ncbi.nlm.nih.gov/29262125/ [Accessed 29 April 2021].

Rose, N. (1999a) *Governing the Soul: The Shaping of the Private Self* (2nd edn), London: Taylor & Francis/Routledge.

Rose, N. (1999b) *Powers of Freedom: Reframing Political Thought*, Cambridge: Cambridge University Press.

Rose, N. (2007) *The Politics of Life Itself: Biomedicine, Power and Subjectivity in the Twenty-First Century*, Oxford: Princeton University Press.

Rose, N. (2013) 'The human sciences in a biological age', *Theory, Culture & Society*, 30(1): 3–34.

Rose, N. (2016) 'Reading the human brain: how the mind became legible', *Body and Society*, 22(2): 140–177.

Rose, N. and Novas, C. (2005) 'Biological citizenship', in A. Ong and S. Collier (eds) *Global Assemblages: Technology, Politics and Ethics as Anthropological Problems*, Malden: Blackwell, 439–463.

Rose, N., O'Malley, P. and Valverde, M. (2006) 'Governmentality', *Annual Review Law Society*, 2: 83–104.

Rotter, J.B. and Rafferty, J.E. (1950) *The Rotter Incomplete Sentences Blank Manual: College Form*, New York: Psychological Corp.

Rozin, P., Scott, S., Dingley, M., Urbanek, J., Hong, J. and Kaltenbach, M. (2011) 'Nudge to nobesity I: minor changes in accessibility decrease food intake', *Journal of the Society for Judgement and Decision Making*, 6(4): 323–332.

Ruckenstein, M. (2014) 'Visualized and interacted life: personal analytics and engagements with data doubles', *Societies*, 4(1): 68–84.

Ruckenstein, M. (2017) 'Digital consumption', in M. Keller, B. Halkier, T.A. Wilska and M. Truninger (eds) *Routledge Handbook of Consumption*, London: Routledge, 466–476.

Ruckenstein, M. and Pantzar, M. (2015) 'Datafied life: techno-anthropology as a site for exploration and experimentation', *Techne*, 19(2): 191–210.

Ruckenstein, M. and Pantzar, M. (2017) 'Beyond the quantified self: thematic exploration of a dataistic paradigm', *New Media & Society*, 19(3): 401–418.

Ruckenstein, M. and Schüll, N.D. (2017) 'The datafication of health', *Annual Review of Anthropology*, 46: 261–278.

Ruckenstein, M. and Kristensen, D.B. (2018) 'Co-evolving with self-tracking technologies', *New Media & Society*, 20(10), doi: https://doi.org/10.1177/1461444818755650.

Ruffino, P. (2018) 'Engagement and the quantified self: uneventful relationships with ghostly companions', in B. Ajana (ed) *Self-Tracking: Empirical and Philosophical Investigations*, Cham: Palgrave Macmillan, 11–26.

Rule, J. (1973) *Private Lives, Public Surveillance*, London: Allen-Lane.

Rule, J., MCadam, D., Stearns, L. and Uglow, D. (1980) *The Politics of Privacy*, New York: New American Library.

Ruppert, E. (2011) 'Population objects: interpassive subjects', *Sociology*, 45(2): 218–233.

Ruppert, E. (2012) 'The governmental topologies of database devices', *Theory, Culture & Society*, 29(4–5): 116–136.

Rymes, B. (2012) 'Recontextualising YouTube: from macro-micro to mass-mediated communicative repertoires', *Anthropology & Education Quarterly*, 43(2): 214–227.

Sabbagh, C., Boyland, E., Hankey, C. and Parrett, A. (2020) 'Analysing Credibility of UK Social Media Influencers' Weight-Management Blogs: A Pilot Study', *International Journal of Environmental Research and Public Health*, 17(23): 9022. doi: 10.3390/ijerph17239022.

Sade-Beck, L. (2004) 'Internet ethnography: online and offline', *International Journal of Qualitative Methods*, 3(2),| Available from: http://www.ualberta.ca/~iiqm/backissues/3_2/html/sadebeck.html [Accessed 12 July 2014].

Sartre, J.P. (1993) *Being and Nothingness*, New York: Washington Square Press.

Saukko, P.M., Reed, M., Britten, N. and Hogarth, S. (2010) 'Negotiating the boundary between medicine and consumer culture: online marketing of nutrigenetic tests', *Social Science and Medicine*, 70(5): 744–753.

Saussure, F. de ([1916]1974) *Course in General Linguistics* (trans W. Baskin), London: Fontana and Collins.

Saussure, F de ([1916]1983) *Course in General Linguistics* (trans R. Harris), London: Duckworth.

Sauter, T. (2014) ' "What's on your mind?" Writing on Facebook as a tool for self-formation', *New Media & Society*, 16(5): 823–839.

Savage, G.C. (2014) 'Chasing the phantoms of public pedagogy: political, popular and concrete publics', in J. Burdick, J.A. Sandlin and M.P. O'Malley (eds) *Problematising Public Pedagogy*, London: Routledge, 79–90.

Savage, M. (2000) *Class Analysis and Social Transformation*, Milton Keynes: Oxford University Press.

Sayer, A. (2011) *Why Things Matter to People: Social Science, Values and Ethical Life*, Cambridge: Cambridge University Press.

Sayette, M.A., Loewenstein, G., Kirchner, T.R. and Travis, T. (2005) 'Effects of smoking urge on temporal cognition', *Psychology of Addictive Behaviours*, 19(1): 88–93.

Scharff, C. (2016) 'The psychic life of neoliberalism: mapping the contours of entrepreneurial subjectivity', *Theory, Culture & Society*, 33: 107–122.

Schilder, P. (1935) *The Image and Appearance of the Human Body*, Oxford: Kegan Paul.

Schreiber, R. (1996) '(Re)defining my self: women's process of recovery from depression', *Qualitative Health Research*, 6(4): 469–491. doi:10.1177/104973239600600402.

Scott, J. (1998) *Seeing Like a State: How Certain Schemes to Improve the Human Condition Have Failed*, New Haven, CT: Yale University Press.

Seale, C. (2003) 'Health and media: an overview', *Sociology of Health & Illness*, 25(6): 513–531.

Shahini, A. (2012) 'Who could be watching you watching your figure? Your boss', NPR.ORG All Tech Considered, 26 December, Available from: http://www.npr.org/blogs/alltechconsidered/2012/12/26/167970303/who-could-be-watching-you-watching-your-figure-your-boss [Accessed 16 October 2021].

Shapin, S. (1994) *A Social History of Truth: Civility and Science in Seventeenth-Century England*, Chicago: University of Chicago Press.

Sharma, A. and Gupta, A. (eds) (2006) *The Anthropology of the State: A Reader*, Malden, MA: Blackwell Publishing..

Sharon, T. (2015) 'Healthy citizenship beyond autonomy and discipline: tactical engagements with genetic testing', *BioSocieties*, 10: 295–316.

Sharon, T. (2016a) 'The Googlization of health research: from disruptive innovation to disruptive ethics', *Personalized Med*icine, 13: 563–574.

Sharon, T. (2016b) 'Self-tracking for health and the quantified self: re-articulating autonomy, solidarity, and authenticity in an age of personalised healthcare', *Philosophy & Technology*, 30: 93–121.

Sharpe, R. (2012) 'Many health apps are based on flimsy science at best and they often do not work', *Wellness Indiana*, 11 December, Available from: http://www.wellnessindiana.org/index.php/article-many-health-apps-are-based-on-flimsy-science-at-best-and-they-often-do-not-work/ [Accessed 10 September 2015].

Shaw, J.M., Mitchell, C.A., Welch, A.J. and Williamson, M.J. (2015) 'Social media used as a health intervention in adolescent health: A systematic review of the literature', *Digital Health*, 1: 1–10.

Sherman, J. (2016) 'Data in the age of digital reproduction: reading the quantified self through Walter Benjamin', in D. Nafus (ed) *Quantified: Biosensing Technologies in Everyday Life*, Cambridge, MA: MIT Press, 27–42.

Shifman, L. (2011) 'An anatomy of a YouTube meme', *New Media & Society*, 14(2): 187–203.

Shull, P.B., Jirattigalachote, W., Hunt, M.A., Cutkosky, M.R. and Delp, S. (2014) 'Quantified self and human movement: a review on the clinical impact of wearable sensing and feedback for gait analysis and intervention', *Gait and Posture*, 40(1): 11–19.

Siebers, T. (2010) *Disability Aesthetics*, Ann Arbor: University of Michigan Press.

Silva, A., de Souza, E. and Sutko, D. (2009) *Digital Cityscapes: Merging Digital and Urban Playspaces*, New York and Oxford: Peter Lang.

Silverstein, M. (1979) 'Language structure and linguistic ideology', in P. Clyne, F. William, C. Hanks and C.L. Hofbauer (eds) *The Elements: A Parasession on Linguistic Units and Levels*, Chicago: Chicago Linguistic Society, 193–247.

Silverstein, M. (2003) 'Indexical order and the dialectics of sociolinguistic life', *Language and Communication*, 23(3–4): 193–229.

Simmel, G. (1950) 'The secret and the secret society', in K.H. Wolff (ed and trans) *The Sociology of Georg Simmel*, Glencoe, IL: Free Press, 305–376.

Slater, A. (2016) 'Social media and appearance concerns', Paper presented at Nuffield Council of Bioethics meeting, London, 22 June.

Smith, J. (2008) *Qualitative Psychology: A Practical Guide to Research Methods*, London: SAGE.

Sparkes, A. and Smith, B. (2014) 'Ethical issues in qualitative research', in A. Sparkes and B. Smith (eds), *Qualitative Research Methods in Sport, Exercise and Health: From Process to Product*, London: Routledge, 206–237.

Sparks, M. (2013) 'The changing contexts of health promotion', *Health Promotion International*, 28(2): 153–156.

Spiller, K. et al (2018) 'Data privacy: users' thoughts on quantified self personal data', in B. Ajana (ed) *Self-Tracking: Empirical and Philosophical Investigations*, Cham: Palgrave Macmillan, 111–126.

Spring, B., Moller, A.C. and Coons, M.J. (2012) 'Multiple health behaviours: overview and implications', *Journal of Public Health* (Oxford), 34(Suppl 1): i3–10. doi: 10.1093/pubmed/fdr111.

Srivastava, S.C., Chandra, S. and Shirish, A. (2015) 'Technostress creators and job outcomes: theorising the moderating influence of personality traits', *Information Systems Journal*, 25(4): 355–401.

Srnicek, N. (2017) *Platform Capitalism*, Vancouver: John Wiley & Sons.

Starr, P. (1982) *The Social Transformation of American Medicine*, New York: Basic Books.

Statistica (2021) 'Global digital health market size in 2019 and a forecast for 2026', Available from: https://www.statista.com/statistics/1092869/global-digital-health-market-size-forecast/ [Accessed 29 April 2021].

Steenackers, K., Cassady, B., Brengman, M. and Willems, K. (2016) 'Measuring Facebook addiction among adults: validating the Bergen Facebook addiction scale in a non-student sample', *Journal of Behavioural Addictions*, 5: 41–47.

Sternberg, R. (1998) 'Styles of thinking and learning', *Canadian Journal of School Psychology*, 13(2): 15–40.

Stevens, C.J. and Bryan, A.D. (2012) 'Rebranding exercise: there's an app for that', *American Journal of Health Promotion*, 27(2): 69–70.

Strategy Analytics (2012) 'Worldwide smartphone population tops 1 billion in Q3 2012', Strategy Analytics, Available from: http://blogs.strategyanalytics.com/WDS/post/2012/10/17/Worldwide-Smartphone- Population-Tops-1-Billion-in-Q3–2012.aspx [Accessed 12 June 2015].

Strathern, M. (1999) *Property, Substance, and Effect: Anthropological Essays on Persons and Things*, London: Athlone Press.

Strathern, M. (ed) (2000) *Audit Culture: Anthropological Studies in Accountability, Ethics and the Academy*, London: Routledge.

Strathern, M. (2005) *Partial Connections*, Lanham, MD: Rowman & Littlefield and AltaMira Press.

Sunderland, J. (2004) *Gendered Discourses*, Basingstoke and New York: Palgrave Macmillan.

Sunstein, C.R. and Thaler, R.H. (2003) 'Libertarian paternalism is not an oxymoron', *The University of Chicago Law Review*, 70(4): 1159–1202.

Swan, M. (2009) 'Emerging patient-driven health care models: an examination of health social networks, consumer personalized medicine and quantified self-tracking', *International Journal of Environmental Research and Public Health*, 6(2): 492–525.

Swan, M. (2012a) 'Health 2050: the realization of personalized medicine through crowdsourcing, the quantified self, and the participatory biocitizen', *Journal of Personalized Medicine*, 2(3): 93–118.

Swan, M. (2012b) 'Sensor mania! The internet of things, wearable computing, objective metrics, and the quantified self 2.0', *Journal of Sensor and Actuator Networks*, 1(3): 217–253.

Swan, M. (2013) 'The quantified self: fundamental disruption in big data science and biological discovery', *Big Data*, 1(2): 85–99.

Swist, T., Collin, P., McCormack, J. and Third, A. (2015) 'Social media and the wellbeing of children and young people: a literature review', Perth, Western Australia, Prepared for the Commissioner for Children and Young People, Western Australia.

Syvertsen, T. and Enli, G. (2020) 'Digital detox: m3edia resistance and the promise of authenticity', *Convergence*, 26(5–6), 1269–1283. https://doi.org/10.1177/1354856519847325.

Syvertsen, T., Mjøs, O., Moe, H. and Enli, G. (2014) *The Media Welfare State: Nordic Media in the Digital Era*, Ann Arbor: University of Michigan Press.

Takahashi, T., Oono, H. and Radford, M.H.B. (2008) 'Psychophysics of time perception and intertemporal choice models', *Physica A: Statistical Mechanics and Its Applications*, 387(8–9): 2066–2074.

Talbot, V.C., Gavin, J., Steen, V.T. and Morey, Y. (2017) 'A content analysis of thinspiration, fitspiration, and bonespiration imagery on social media', *Journal of Eating Disorders*, 5(40), doi: 10.1186/s40337-017-0170-2.

Taleb, J. (2012) 'Self quantification of health and fitness', *Journal of the American College of Cardiology*, 60(16): 1574–1575.

Tamburrini, G. and Datteri, E. (2009) 'Ethical reflections on health care robotics', in R. Capurro (ed) *Ethics and Robotics*, Amsterdam: IOS Press, 35–48.

Tapscott, D. and Williams, A.D. (2008) *Wikinomics: How Mass Collaboration Changes Everything*, London: Portfolio.

Tarantino, M. and Tosoni, S. (2013) 'Introduction: beyond the centrality of media and the centrality of space', *First Monday*, 18(11), Available from: http://firstmonday.org/ojs/index.php/ fm/article/view/4953 [Accessed 7 February 2022].

Temperton, J. (2018) 'How to check if your Facebook data was shared with Cambridge Analytica', *Wired*, 10 April, Available from: http://www.wired.co.uk/article/how-to-check-if-your-facebook-data-was-shared-with-cambridge-analytica [Accessed 1 June 2018].

Terranova, T. (2000) 'Free labor: producing culture for the digital economy', *Social Text*, 18(2): 33–58.

Thacker, E. (2003) 'What is biomedia?', *Configurations*, 11(1): 47–79.

Thaler, C. and Sunstein, R. (2009) *Nudge: Improving Decisions about Health, Wealth and Happiness*, London: Penguin.

The Medical Futurist (2017) 'The top 15 examples of gamification in healthcare', 20 July. Available from: https://medicalfuturist.com/top-examples-of-gamification-in-healthcare/ [Accessed: 23 February 2023].

Thiel-Stern, K. (2012) 'Beyond the active audience exploring new media audiences and the limits of cultural production', in Valdivia, A.N. (ed) *The International Encyclopedia of Media Studies*, New York: John Wiley.

Thoermer, S. (2012) 'Quantified self – Das eigene Leben messbar machen', Available from: http://www.wirtschafts-news.org/news/article/quantified- self-das-eigene-leben-messbar-machen.html [Accessed 14 June 2015].

Thumin, N. (2012) *Self-Representation and Digital Culture*, Basingstoke: Palgrave Macmillan.

Tifentale, A. and Manovich, L. (2014) 'Selfiecity: exploring photography and self-fashioning in social media'. Available from: http://manovich.net/content/04-projects/086-selfiecity-exploring/selfiecity_chapter.pdf [Accessed 22 February 2023].

Tiggemann, M. (2011) 'Sociocultural perspectives on human appearance and body image', in T.F. Cash and L. Smolak (eds) *Body Image: A Handbook of Science, Practice, and Prevention* (2nd edn), New York: Guilford Press, 12–19.

Till, C. (2014) 'Exercise as labour: quantified self and the transformation of exercise into labour', *Societies*, 4(3): 446–462.

Till, C. (2018) 'Self-tracking as the mobilisation of the social for capital accumulation', in B. Ajana (ed), *Self-Tracking: Empirical and Philosophical Investigations*, Cham: Palgrave Macmillan, 77–92.

Toffler, A. (1980) *The Third Wave*, New York: William Morrow.

Topol, E. (2012) *The Creative Destruction of Medicine: How the Digital Revolution Will Create Better Health Care*, New York: Basic Books.

Torpey, J. (2007) 'Through thick and thin: surveillance after 9/11', *Contemporary Sociology*, 36(2): 116–119.

Townsend, A. (2013) *Smart Cities: Big Data, Civic Hackers, and the Quest for a New Utopia*, New York: W.W. Norton and Company.

Tritter, J.Q. (2009) 'Revolution or evolution: the challenges of conceptualizing patient and public involvement in a consumerist world', *Health Expectations*, 12(3): 275–287.

Trottier, D. (2012) *Social Media as Surveillance: Rethinking Visibility in a Converging World*, London: Routledge.

Tufecki, Z. (2008) 'Can you see me now? Audience and disclosure regulation in online social network sites', *Bulletin of Science, Technology and Society*, 28(1): 20–36.

Turel, O. (2015) 'Quitting the use of a habituated hedonic information system: a theoretical model and empirical examination of Facebook users', *European Journal of Information Systems*, 24(4): 431–446.

Turel, O., He, Q., Xue, G., Xiao, L. and Bechara, A. (2017) 'Examination of neural systems subserving Facebook "addiction"', *Psychological Reports NCBI*, 115(3): 675–695.

Turel, O., Mouttapa, M. and Donato, E. (2015) 'Preventing problematic Internet use through video-based interventions: a theoretical model and empirical test', *Behaviour & Information Technology*, 34: 349–362. doi:10.1080/0144929x.2014.936041.

Turel, O. and Qahri-Saremi, H. (2016) 'Problematic use of social networking sites: antecedents and consequence from a dual-system theory perspective', *Journal of Management Information Systems*, 33(4): 1087–1116.

Turel, O., Romashkin, A. and Morrison, K.M. (2016) 'Health outcomes of information system use lifestyles among adolescents: videogame addiction, sleep curtailment and cardio-metabolic deficiencies', *PLoS ONE*, 11: e0154764, doi: 10.1371/journal.pone.0154764.

Turel, O. and Serenko, A. (2012) 'The benefits and dangers of enjoyment with social networking websites', *European Journal of Information Systems*, 21(5): 512–528.

Turel, O., Serenko, A. and Giles, P. (2011) 'Integrating technology addiction and use: an empirical investigation of online auction sites', *MIS Quarterly*, 35(4): 1043–1061.

Turkle, S. (2011) *Alone Together: Why We Expect More from Technology and Less from Each Other*, New York: Basic Books.

Turkle, S. (2015) *Reclaiming Conversation: The Power of Talk in a Digital Age*, New York: Penguin.

UK Government (2021) 'NHS Test and Trace: what to do if you are contacted', Available from: https://www.gov.uk/guidance/nhs-test-and-trace-how-it-works [Accessed 29 April 2021].

Upshur, R. (2002) 'Principles for the justification of public health intervention', *Public Health*, 93(2): 101–103.

Urry, J. and Elliot, J. (2010) *Mobile Lives*, London: Routledge.

Ursell, G. (2000) 'Television production: issues of exploitation, commodification and subjectivity in UK television labour markets', *Media, Culture & Society*, 22(6): 805–882.

Vaithianathan, R., Ryan, M., Anchugina, N., Selvey, L., Dare, T. and Brown, A. (2020) 'Digital contact tracing for Covid-19: A primer for policymakers', Centre for Social Data Analytics: Auckland University of Technology & The University of Queensland, Available from: issr.uq.edu.au/files/14448/PolicyPrimer.pdf [Accessed 16 March 2023].

Vallgårda, S. (2012) 'Nudge: a new and better way to improve health?', *Health Policy*, 104(2): 200–203. doi: 10.1016/j.healthpol.2011.10.013.

Valtorta, N.K. et al (2016) 'Loneliness and social isolation as risk factors for coronary heart disease and stroke: systematic review and meta-analysis of longitudinal observational studies', *Heart (British Cardiac Society)*, 102(13): 1009–1016, doi: 10.1136/heartjnl-2015-308790.

Van der Mars, H. (1989) 'Observer reliability: issues and procedures', in P.W. Darst, D.B. Zakrajsek and V.H. Mancini (eds) *Analysing Physical Education and Sport Instruction* (2nd edn), Champaign, IL: Human Kinetics, 53–80.

Van der Schaaf, P. and Oderwald, A. (1999) *Chronisch zieken over ervaringsdeskundigheid* [The chronically Ill about experiential expertise], Amsterdam: Vrije Universiteit Amsterdam.

Van der Tuin, I. and Dolphijn, R. (2010) 'The transversality of new materialism', *Women: A Cultural Review*, 21(2): 153–171.

van Dijck, J. (2013a) '"You have one identity": performing the self on Facebook and LinkedIn', *Media, Culture & Society*, 35(2): 199–215.

van Dijck, J. (2013b) *The Culture of Connectivity: A Critical History of Social Media*, Oxford: Oxford University Press.

van Dijck, J. (2014) 'Datafication, dataism and dataveillance: big data between scientific paradigm and ideology', *Surveillance and Society*, 12(2): 197–208.

van Dijck, T. (2004) 'Critical discourse analysis', in D. Schiffrin, D. Tannen and H.E. Hamilton (eds) *The Handbook of Discourse Analysis*, Oxford: Blackwell, 352–371.

van Maanen, J. (1988) *Tales of the Field*, Chicago: The University of Chicago Press.

Van Remoortel, H. et al (2012) 'Validity of activity monitors in health and chronic disease: a systematic review', *International Journal of Behavioral Nutrition and Physical Activity*, 9: 84. Available from: http://www.ijbnpa.org/content/9/1/84 [Accessed 5 October 2021].

Varis, P. (2014) 'Digital ethnography', Tilburg Papers in Cultural Studies 104, Available from: https://www.tilburguniversity.edu/upload/c428e18c-935f-4d12–8afb-652e19899a30_TPCS_104_Varis.pdf [Accessed 1 May 2022].

Vaz, P. and Bruno, F. (2003) 'Types of self-surveillance: from abnormality to individuals "at risk"', *Surveillance & Society*, 1(3): 272–291.

Verbeek, P.P. (2005) *What Things Do: Philosophical Reflections on Technology, Agency, and Design*, University Park: The Pennsylvania State University Press.

Verbeek, P.P. (2011) *Moralizing Technology: Understanding and Designing the Morality of Things*, London: The University of Chicago Press.

Verbrugge, L. (1980) 'Sex differences in complaints and diagnoses', *Journal of Behavioural Medicine*, 3(4): 327–355.

Vincent, B.B. (2016) 'From self-organization to self-assembly: a new materialism?' *History and Philosophy of the Life Sciences*, 38(3): 1. doi: 10.1007/s40656-016-0108-z.

Viseu, A. and Suchman, L. (2010) 'Wearable augmentations', in J. Edwards, P. Harvey and P. Wade (eds) *Technologized Images, Technologized Bodies: Anthropological Approaches to a New Politics of Vision*, Oxford and New York: Berghahn Books, 161–184.

Wajcman, J. (2014) *Pressed for Time: The Acceleration of Life in Digital Capitalism*, Chicago: The University of Chicago Press.

Wakefield, A. and Fleming, J. (2009) *The Sage Dictionary of Policing*, London: SAGE.

Waldby, C. (2000) 'Virtual anatomy: from the body in the text to the body on the screen', *Journal of Medical Humanities*, 21(2): 85–107.

Walker-Rettberg, J. (2015) *Seeing Ourselves through Technology: How We Use Selfies, Blogs and Wearable Devices to See and Shape Ourselves*, Basingstoke: Palgrave Macmillan.

Wallace, P. (1999) *The Psychology of the Internet*, New York: Cambridge University Press.

Walsh, M. and Baker, S.A. (2020) 'Clean eating and Instagram: purity, defilement and the idealisation of food', *Food, Culture, and Society*, 23(5): 570–588. doi: 10.1080/15528014.2020.1806636.

Waltz, E. (2012) 'How I quantified myself', *Institute of Electrical and Electronics Engineers (IEEE) Spectrum*, 30 August, Available from: https://spectrum.ieee.org/biomedical/devices/how-i-quantified-myself [Accessed 1 May 2020].

Wang, X. (2016) *How the World Changed Social Media*, London: UCL Press.

Warin, M. (2011) 'Foucault's progeny: Jamie Oliver and the art of governing obesity', *Social Theory & Health*, 9(1): 24–40.

Wartella, E., Rideout, V., Montague, H., Beaudoin-Ryan, L. and Lauricella, A. (2016) 'Teens, health, and technology: a national survey', *Media and Communication*, 4(3): 13–23.

Warzel, C. (2019) 'All your data is health data: and big tech has it all', *New York Times*, 13 August, Available from: https://www.nytimes.com/2019/08/13/opinion/health-data.html [Accessed 29 April 2021].

Webb, L. and Quennerstedt, M. (2010) 'Risky bodies: health surveillance and teachers' embodiment of health', *International Journal of Qualitative Studies in Education*, 23(7): 785–802.

Weber, M. (1978) *Economy and Society: An Outline of Interpretive Sociology* (Vol. 2), Berkeley: University of California Press.

Wei, R. (2013) 'Mobile media: coming of age with a big splash', *Mobile Media & Communication*, 46(1): 39–50.

Weintraub, K. (2013) 'Quantified self: the tech-based route to a better life?', *BBC Future*, 3 January, Available from: http://www.bbc.com/future/story/20130102-self-track-route-to-a-better-life [Accessed 16 October 2020].
Wellman, B. (2003) 'Sousveillance: inventing and using wearable computing devices for data collection in surveillance environments', *Surveillance & Society*, 1(3): 331–355.
Westin, A. (1967) *Privacy and Freedom*, New York: Columbia University Press.
Whitson, J. and Haggerty, K.D. (2008) 'Identity theft and the care of the virtual self', *Economy and Society*, 37(4): 572–594.
Whitson, J.R. (2013) 'Gaming the quantified self', *Surveillance & Society*, 11(1/2): 163–176.
Williams, R. (1981) *Culture*, London: Fontana.
Williams, R. (1990) *Television, Technology & Cultural Form*, London: Routledge.
Williams, R. and Miller, D. (1998) 'Producing AIDS news', in D. Miller, J. Kitzinger, K. Williams and P. Beharrell (eds) *The Circuits of Mass Communication*, London: SAGE, 147–166.
Willig, C. (2001) *Introducing Qualitative Research in Psychology: Adventures on Theory and Method*, Buckingham and Philadelphia: Open University Press.
Willig, C. (2003) 'Discourse analysis', in Smith, J.A. (ed) *Qualitative Psychology: A Practical Guide to Methods*, London: SAGE, 159–183.
Wilson, A.G. et al (2015) 'Predictors of delay discounting among smokers: education level and a utility measure of cigarette reinforcement efficacy are better predictors than demographics, smoking characteristics, executive functioning, impulsivity, or time perception', *Journal of Addictive Behaviours*, 45: 124–133.
Wilson, R.S. et al (2007) 'Loneliness and risk of Alzheimer disease', *Archives of General Psychiatry*, 64(2): 234–240, doi: 10.1001/archpsyc.64.2.234.
Winch, A. (2013) *Girlfriends and Postfeminist Sisterhood*, Basingstoke: Palgrave Macmillan.
Winnicott, D.W. (1971) *Playing and Reality*, London: Tavistock Publications.
Wittmann, M. and Paulus, M.P. (2008) 'Decision making, impulsivity and time perception', *Trends in Cognitive Sciences*, 12(1): 7–12.
Wittmann, M., Leland, D.S. and Paulus, M.P. (2006) 'The neurobiology of inter-temporal reward selection: fMRI activation of insular cortex and striaturn during delay discounting', *Biological Psychiatry*, 59(8): 166S–167S.
Wodak, R. and Meyer, M. (2009) *Methods of Critical Discourse Analysis: History, Theory and Methodology*, London: SAGE.
Wolf, E.J., Harrington, K.M., Clark, S.L. and Miller, M.W. (2013) 'Sample size requirements for structural equation models: An evaluation of power, bias, and solution propriety', *Educational and Psychological Measurement*, 73(6), 913–934.
Wolf, G. (2009) 'The social memex – Mark Carranza's memory experiment', Quantified Self, Available from: https://quantifiedself.com/blog/the-social-memex/ Accessed February 21 2023.

Wolf, G. (2010) 'The data-driven life', *New York Times*, 28 April, Available from: http://www.nytimes.com/2010/05/02/magazine/02self-measurement-t.html?_r=3&ref=magazine&pagewanted=all [Accessed 13 June 2020].

Wolf, G. and Kelly, K. (2010) 'The data-driven life', *The New York Times*. Available from: https://www.nytimes.com/2010/05/02/magazine/02self-measurement-t.html [Accessed 23 February 2023].

World Health Organization (2011) *Mhealth: New Horizons for Health through Technologies. Global Observatory Series, 3*, Geneva: World Health Organisation, Available from: http://www.who.int/goe/publications/goe_mhealth_web.pdf [Accessed 1 June 2018].

World Health Organization (2021) World Health Organisation main page, Available from: https://www.who.int/ [Accessed 29 April 2021].

World Health Organization World Health Report (2008) 'Primary Health Care (now more than ever)', Geneva, Available from: http://www.who.int/whr/2008/en/ [Accessed 1 June 2018].

Wright, J. and Harwood, V. (2009) *Biopolitics and the 'Obesity Epidemic': Governing Bodies*, New York: Routledge.

Yee, N. and Bailenson, J. (2007) 'The Proteus Effect: the effect of transformed self-representation on behavior', *Human Communication Research*, 33: 271–290.

Yeung, K. (2009) 'Towards an understanding of regulation by design', in R. Brownsword and K. Yeung (eds) *Regulating Technologies*, Oxford: Hart Publishing, 79–80.

Yeung, K. and Dixon-Woods, M. (2010) 'Design-based regulation and patient safety: a regulatory studies perspective', *Social Science Medicine*, 71(3): 502–509.

Zhao, S., Grasmuck, S. and Martin, J. (2008) 'Identity construction on Facebook: digital empowerment in anchored relationships', *Computers in Human Behaviour*, 24: 1816–1836.

Zichermann, G. and Cunningham, C. (2011) *Gamification by Design: Implementing Game Mechanics in Web and Mobile Apps*, Sebastopol: O'Reilly Media.

Ziebland, S. and Wyke, S. (2012) 'Health and illness in a connected world: how might sharing experiences on the internet affect people's health?' *Milbank Q*. 90(2): 219–249.

Zimmerman, D. and Weider, D.L. (1977) 'Diary-interview method', *Urban Life*, 5(4): 479–498.

Zuboff, S. (2015) 'Big other: surveillance capitalism and the prospects of an information civilization', *Journal of Information Technology*, 30: 75–89.

Zuboff, S. (2019) *The Age of Surveillance Capitalism: The Fight for a Human Future at the New Frontier of Power*, London: Profile Books.

Zuckerberg, M. (2012) in Van Dijck, J. (2013) '"You have one identity": performing the self on Facebook and LinkedIn', *Media, Culture and Society*, 35(2): 199.

Index

References to figures appear in *italic* type.

E

I

J

K

L

M

N